OCEAN OF STREAMS

SHIATSU

MERIDIANS, TSUBOS AND THEORETICAL IMPRESSIONS

Colouring Sections

VEET JOHN ALLAN, MRSS

TO GORAK AND FRIENDS

This edition published by:

Om Shiatsu Centre
Administration
10 Kipps Avenue
AIRDRIE
ML6 0JG

First Printing 1994
Reprinted 1995

ISBN : 0 9523976 09

This book is not designed to diagnose, prescribe or treat any ailment without adequate professional training nor is it intended in any way as a replacement for medical consultation.

ACKNOWLEDGEMENTS

This project would not have been realised without the encouragement and ideas I have received from my teachers, students and fellow practitioners. I am particularly indebted to the following:

- **Elaine Liechti** for presenting the wider view of Chinese Medicine and providing me with the opportunity to teach Shiatsu in the first place.

- **Shinmei Kishi** who, when asked by a student "What about the Zen Shiatsu Meridian Chart?" replied "Ask Masunaga!"

- **Pauline Sasaki** and **Clifford Andrews** whose earlier developments on Masunaga's work and clear teaching gave me initial guidance and inspiration.

- **Sada Stewart** for the typescript and helping me with the editing and overall layout. Due to her patience with my never ending additions this project is now realised.

- **Vanya Turnbull** for assisting me in various classes and suggesting the drawings and theoretical studies be put into print.

Finally I would like to thank my Parents for providing me with space where the project could be finalised, and my friend Jila whose love and support ensured that it was.

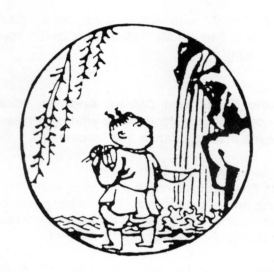

PREFACE

I originally devised the bare bones of this project in order to clearly present the Zen Shiatsu meridian system as a central focus alongside those of Traditional Chinese Medicine, Western anatomy, physiology and psychology to students at the Om Shiatsu Centre, Glasgow over the past two years.

Fundamentally this work follows the guidelines of the baseline curriculum set by the Shiatsu Society for teaching students towards practitioner status in this country. However, my interpretation of the Zen Shiatsu system does differ in parts from the original works of its founder the late Shizuto Masunaga of Japan. This is simply due to modern developments of this work which I have been taught and my current perception in practice.

As far as I know, this is the first attempt at detailing and illustrating a Zen Shiatsu based system in relation to the aforementioned ones. It has proved difficult in various areas as the original charts and book sources consulted do contain errors of both artistic and technical origin. Subsequently it is my hope that by self colouring the illustrations and augmenting them with the theoretical sections, the student or practitioner will come into contact with these aspects and in doing so, provide themselves with a pictorial guide of where the various systems may or may not be compatible.

6 June 1994   **Veet John Allan, MRSS**

HOW TO USE THIS BOOK

There are six main sections, five of which are headed by an Element from Traditional Chinese Medicine. These are then subdivided to contain the relevant Elemental and Zen Shiatsu meridian correspondences in addition to Zang Fu (organ)/Zen Shiatsu (meridian) functions, Residential Tsubo Studies and the Meridian Illustrations. The final section contains an illustrated study of all meridians in key body areas or zones and contains the tsubos of the Conception Vessel and Governing Vessel.

All illustrations, including the Five Element symbols, are designed for self colouring. Although you may prefer to colour the meridians only, it is also possible to include the musco-skeletal system if a full colour image is required. To obtain the best results I recommend the use of eleven felt tip pens, Berol Colourpens R11 & C11 for the meridians/tsubos and two coloured pencils (Berol Verithin) for the muscles/bones.

The colour for each meridian relates to the dominant element and is further differentiated into lighter or darker shades according to the yin or yang status respectively. Please note that it is best to colour the relevant traditional tsubos first as some of them appear on other meridians within the Zen Shiatsu system. A full legend is provided as a guide for self colouring and referencing.

To preserve the quality of the drawings it is suggested that you insert a thicker page directly behind the page you are colouring.

COLOUR LEGEND AND REFERENCE

FIVE ELEMENTS

Water	Aqua Blue
Wood	Light Green
Fire	Red
Earth	Yellow
Metal	White

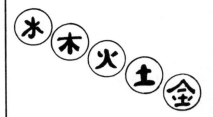

MERIDIAN/TSUBO SYSTEMS

Yin Meridian

Yang Meridian

Tsubo recommended by Shiatsu Society for study
Traditional meridian tsubo on Zen Shiatsu meridian e.g. TH2 on Stomach meridian
Meridian enters internal pathway
Extra - Traditional Meridial Tsubo

CV - Conception Vessel
GV - Governing Vessel

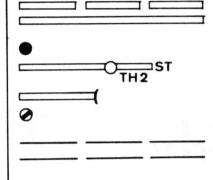

Meridian & Traditional Tsubo Colours/Index

LU	=	Lung	White
LI	=	Large Intestine	Light Grey
ST	=	Stomach	Brown
SP	=	Spleen (Pancreas)	Yellow
HT	=	Heart	Pink
SI	=	Small Intestine	Red
BL	=	Bladder	Dark Blue
KD	=	Kidney	Aqua Blue
HG	=	Heart Governor	Orange
TH	=	Triple Heater	Purple
GB	=	Gall Bladder	Dark Green
LV	=	Liver	Light Green

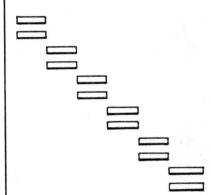

DIAGNOSTIC ZONES (ZEN SHIATSU)

Hara (abdomen) or Back diagnostic zone

** For overall clarity it is best these zones are coloured around the inside perimeter only. The only exceptions are the schematic illustrations of the meridian pairs (Sections 1-5) and the complete Hara/Back (Section 6).
The related meridian colour can be used on all of the above. **

MUSCO-SKELETAL SYSTEM

Muscles	= light 'dusting'	Rose 52
Tendons	=	White
Bones	= light 'dusting'	Yellow Ochre 89

MEASUREMENT

Oriental anatomical inch:

Sun (Japanese)	]	Scarlet Red 55
Cun (Chinese)	]	

Common unit derived from the thumb width of the person being treated.

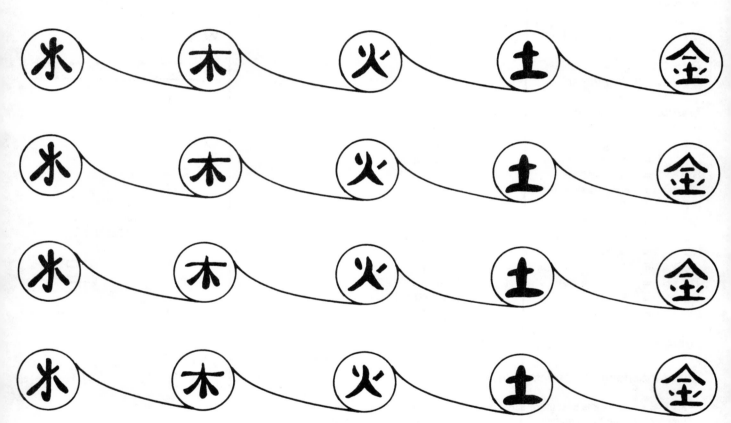

CONTENTS

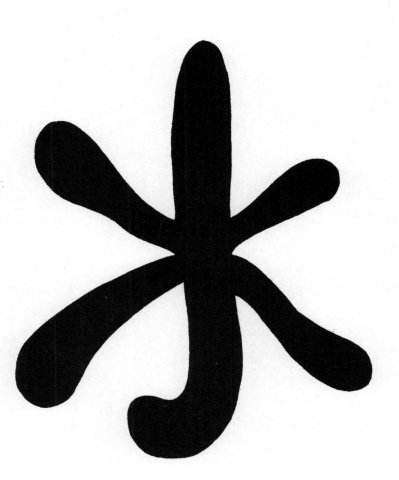

THE FIVE ELEMENT CORRESPONDENCES

FACULTY

Spiritual	Essence	JING
	Willpower	ZHI
Genetic	Conception	
Cycle	Storage	
Yin/Yang	Utmost Yin	
Quality	Floating	

ENVIRONMENTAL

Season	Winter
Climate	Cold
Direction	North
Part of Day	Nightime
	12am-5am
Colour	Black, Blue

BODY

Organ	Yin	Kidney
	Yang	Bladder
Tissue		Marrow, Bones
Sense Organ		Ears
Senses		Hearing
Branch		Head Hair
Skin Colour		Black, Blue
Odour		Putrid
Fluid		Watery Saliva
		Urine

EMOTIONAL

Emotion	Fear
	Courage
Sound, Voice	Groaning
	Humming
Action	Trembling

FOOD

Animal	Pig, Fish
Fruit	Chestnut
Grain	Beans
Vegetable	Leek
	Root Plants
Taste	Salty

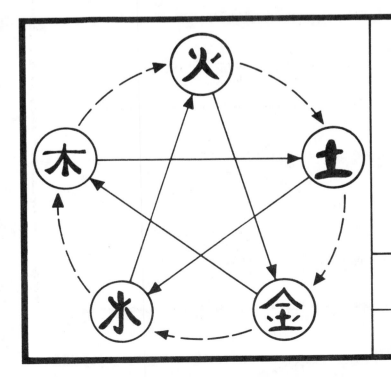

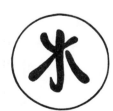

WATER

ZEN SHIATSU MERIDIAN CORRESPONDENCES

BLADDER MERIDIAN
PAN KUNG ching

FACULTY		
	Spiritual Input	: ZHI via Kidney Meridian
	Functions via	: Survival
	Represents	: Fluidity
	Supplemented by	: Nervous Communication
	Realised via	: Understanding
	Dominant Zone	: Back
	Embryological Layer	: Endoderm
	Meridian Nature	: Yang
	Tuning Time	: 3pm - 5pm

ANATOMY & PHYSIOLOGY		
	Medulla Oblongata	] Autonomic Nervous System
	Cerebellum	] (ANS)
	Spinal Cord	] Information, Movement, Balance
	Eyes	] Response
	Hypothalamus	] Hormonal System
	Pituitary Gland	] Reproductive System
	Uterus	]
	Kidneys	] Urinary System
	Ureters	] Fluid Balance
	Bladder	]

PHYSICAL		
	ANS Disorders	Nasal Congestion
	Back & Neck Problems	Nervous Tension/Stress
	Chills - Back/Lower Body	Oedema
	Cramp	Palpitations
	Cystitis	Prostrate Problems
	Distended Lower Hara	Retention of Urine
	Dizziness	Sciatica
	Eye/Vision Problems	Tight Shoulders
	Headaches	Urinary Disorders
	Incontinence	Uterine Problems

PSYCHOLOGICAL		
	Alertness	Overactive
	Anxiety	Oversensitive
	Complaining	Phobias
	Desire	Restful
	Easily Startled	Seeking Balanced Lifestyle
	Evasive	Stress
	Fear	Sudden Tiredness
	Fretful	Suspicious Nature
	Issues of Character	Unnecessary Worry
	Neurotic	Weighing Up Situation

ZEN SHIATSU MERIDIAN CORRESPONDENCES

KIDNEY MERIDIAN
SHEN ching

FACULTY		
	Spiritual Input	: ZHI, Willpower
	Functions via	: Survival
	Represents	: Synchronisation
	Supplemented by	: Hormonal Communication
	Realised via	: Responding
	Dominant Zone	: Back
	Embryological Layer	: Endoderm
	Meridian Nature	: Yin
	Tuning Time	: 5pm - 7pm

ANATOMY & PHYSIOLOGY		
	Cerebrum	] Endocrine Gland System (EGS)
	Hypothalamus	] Hormonal System
	Pituitary Gland	] Information, Movement, Balance
	Ears	] Response
	Adrenal Glands	] Reproductive Response
	Kidneys	] Fluid Metabolism
	Ureters	] Urinary System
	Teeth	] Skeletal System
	Spine	]
	Bones	]
	Hair	] Integumentary System

PHYSICAL		
	Back Pain	Inflammation of Throat
	Baldness, Hair Loss	Lack of Body Tone
	Blood Problems	Oedema
	Coldness in Lower Body	Osteoporosis
	Darkness around Eyes	Poor Circulation
	Earache & Toothache	Premature Ageing
	Head Heaviness	Reproductive Problems
	Hearing Problems	Respiratory Disorders
	Hormonal Deficiency	Tension in Abdominal Muscles
	Impotence, Frigidity	Urinary Disorders, inc Stones

PSYCHOLOGICAL		
	Anxiety	Inability to Complete Things
	Apprehensive	Lack of Composure
	Continual Stress	Lack of Drive
	Easily Startled	Listening Situations
	Easy Going	Overactiveness
	Excessive Fear	Phobias
	Exhaustion	Self Hate
	Feels Alone	Timidity
	Guilt	Timing
	How to Co-ordinate	Working All the Time

FUNCTIONAL SYSTEM	MERIDIAN / ORGAN FUNCTIONS IN ORIENTAL MEDICINE	

ZANGFU	KIDNEYS SHEN Stores Essence (JING) Rules reproduction and growth Produces Marrow, fills Brain, controls Bones Foundation of Yin/Yang Governs Water Controls reception of Ki Opens into the Ears Manifests in Head Hair Houses Willpower (ZHI)	BLADDER PANG GUANG Receives and excretes Urine
IMAGE	Strong and **Capable Ministers** from whom Technical Ability and Expertise is derived	**Governor** of the State Capital from where the Water flows
CHINESE GOVT POST	DIRECTOR	REGIONAL MANAGER

ZEN SHIATSU	KIDNEY Meridian SHEN ching Governs Endocrine System (Glands and Hormones) Responds to Stress via Adrenal Glands Responds to Reproductive Drive via Sex Hormones Purifies the Blood Regulates Urine formation	BLADDER Meridian P'AN KUNG ching Governs Autonomic Nervous System (ANS) Relates to Pituitary Gland and KD Hormonal System Controls Reproductive System and the Uterus Regulates elimination of Body Fluids and Urine via purification of Ki
BASIC	**Controls Energy to Body for instinctive Survival**	**Monitors and purifies Energy for instinctive Survival**
SPECIFIC	STAY OR GO HORMONAL COMMUNICATION	REST OR ACTIVITY NERVOUS COMMUNICATION
GENERAL	IMPETUS	

IDENTIFICATION	ACTION	INDICATIONS
BL 1 Jingming EYE BRIGHTNESS Near the medial ORBITAL BORDER, lateral and 0.1 SUN superior to the INNER CANTHUS GV, SI, TH, ST & BL MEETING POINT **** Moxibustion is contraindicated ****	Expels Exterior Wind Clears Heat	All eye problems including red, painful, swollen and dry eyes Frontal and occipital headaches Dizziness, colour or night blindness Pituitary, Hypothalamus and Pineal gland problems
BL 2 Zanzhu GATHERING BAMBOO In the hollow at the medial end of the EYEBROW in the SUPRAORBITAL NOTCH	Expels Wind Brightens Eyes Soothes Liver Removes Channel obstructions Clears the Nose	Facial paralysis and tics Trigeminal Neuralgia Red eyes, blurred vision Eye problems where other Liver distortions are present Frontal headaches and pain around or behind eyes Lower back problems Sinusitis, Rhinitis and Hay Fever
BL 10 Tianzhu HEAVENLY PILLAR 1.3 SUN lateral to GV 15 on the lateral border of the TRAPEZIUS muscle SEA OF KI POINT	Expels Interior and Exterior Wind Clears the Brain Brightens the Eyes Removes Channel obstructions	Occipital and vertical type headaches Stiff neck, nasal congestion Memory and concentration problems Dim vision, eye pain Back pain, neck injuries Cold type pain with stiffness
BL 13 Feishu LUNG'S HOLLOW 1.5 SUN lateral to the centre of the SPINE between the 3rd and 4th THORACIC VERTEBRA LUNG YU/SHU or BACK TRANSPORTING POINT	Stimulates the Lung Dispersing/Descending function Clears Interior Heat Tonifies Lung Ki Regulates LU Defensive Ki	Cough due to Exterior pattern Asthma, cough or breathless symptoms due to Interior pattern Acute Heat conditions i.e. high fever, thirst, cough, breathlessness, sticky yellow sputum, restlessness Breathlessness, chest pain, tight chest, neck or back pain Grief or sadness Skin problems, sweating and fever

IDENTIFICATION	ACTION	INDICATIONS
BL 14 Jueyinshu ABSOLUTE YIN HOLLOW 1.5 SUN lateral to the centre of the SPINE between the 4th and 5th THORACIC VERTEBRA HEART CONSTRICTOR YU/SHU or BACK TRANSPORTING POINT	Regulates the Heart Calms the Mind	Heartbeat problems, pain Coronary heart disease Anxiety and restlessness
BL 15 Xinshu HEART'S HOLLOW 1.5 SUN lateral to the centre of the SPINE between the 5th and 6th THORACIC VERTEBRA HEART YU/SHU or BACK TRANSPORTING POINT	Clears Heat Calms the Mind Stimulates the Brain Invigorates the Blood	Nervous anxiety and insomnia Night sweats Heat in palms and soles Excess conditions of the Heart Concentration and memory problems Heart or chest pain due to stasis of blood
BL 16 Dushu GOVERNING HOLLOW 1.5 SUN lateral to the centre of the SPINE between the 6th and 7th THORACIC VERTEBRA GOVERNING VESSEL YU/SHU or BACK TRANSPORTING POINT	Regulates the Heart Invigorates the Blood	Heart or chest pain Removes blood stasis
BL 17 Geshu DIAPHRAGM'S HOLLOW 1.5 SUN lateral to the centre of the SPINE between the 7th and 8th THORACIC VERTEBRA DIAPHRAGM YU/SHU or BACK TRANSPORTING POINT GATHERING POINT FOR BLOOD	Nourishes Blood and Ki c/w direct Moxibustion Invigorates the Blood Removes obstruction from the Diaphragm Pacifies Stomach Ki	Absence of menses Blood deficiency of organs (treat BL 17 c/w relevant YU point) Lethargy Dizziness Blood stasis in organs or any part of the body Chest pain, hiccup, belching Hiccup, belching, nausea and vomiting

IDENTIFICATION	ACTION	INDICATIONS
BL 18 Ganshu LIVER'S HOLLOW 1.5 SUN lateral to the centre of the SPINE between the 9th and 10th THORACIC VERTEBRA LIVER YU/SHU or BACK TRANSPORTING POINT	Moves stagnant Ki	Distension of epigastrium and hypochondrium Sour regurgitation and nausea
	Resolves Damp Heat	Jaundice and inflammation of the Gall Bladder
	Benefits the Eyes	Poor night vision, blurred eyes Red, painful eyes
	Tonifies Liver Blood	Fatigue Atrophy syndrome (wasting)
BL 19 Danshu GALLBLADDER'S HOLLOW 1.5 SUN lateral to the centre of the SPINE between the 10th and 11th THORACIC VERTEBRA GALL BLADDER YU/SHU or TRANSPORTING POINT	Resolves Damp Heat	Inflammation of Gall Bladder Jaundice Inflammation of Pancreas
	Pacifies Stomach Ki	Nausea, belching, vomiting and heartburn
	Relaxes Diaphragm	Hiccup Full feeling under the diaphragm due to stagnation of Liver Ki
BL 20 Pishu SPLEEN'S HOLLOW 1.5 SUN lateral to the centre of the SPINE between the 11th and 12th THORACIC VERTEBRA SPLEEN YU/SHU or BACK TRANSPORTING POINT	Tonifies Spleen and Stomach	Tiredness, loose stools, no appetite Abdominal distension Prolapse of Stomach or Uterus
	Resolves Damp	Asthma, oedema on torso, dizziness and vertigo
	Nourishes Blood	Anaemia Mental exhaustion Chronic fatigue
BL 21 Weishu STOMACH'S HOLLOW 1.5 SUN lateral to the centre of the SPINE between the 12th THORACIC VERTEBRA and 1st LUMBAR VERTEBRA STOMACH YU/SHU or BACK TRANSPORTING POINT	Tonifies Stomach and Spleen	Loss of appetite Stomach pain, Epigastric pain Pain in the chest or in hypochondriac zone
	Resolves Damp	Asthma, oedema, dizziness and vertigo
	Pacifies Stomach	Belching, hiccup, nausea and vomiting Retention of food causing bloating and regurgitation of food Difficulty swallowing

IDENTIFICATION	ACTION	INDICATIONS
BL 22 Sanjiaoshu TRIPLE HEATER'S HOLLOW 1.5 SUN lateral to the centre of the SPINE between the 1st and 2nd LUMBAR VERTEBRA TRIPLE HEATER YU/SHU or BACK TRANSPORTING POINT	Resolves Dampness Opens Water Passages	Urinary retention, painful urination Oedema of legs Fluid problems in lower torso Kidney stones Lower back pain
BL 23 Shenshu KIDNEY'S HOLLOW 1.5 SUN lateral to the centre of the SPINE between the 2nd and 3rd LUMBAR VERTEBRA KIDNEY YU/SHU or BACK TRANSPORTING POINT **** Do not overstimulate during pregnancy ****	Tonifies Kidneys Nourishes Essence	Chronic fatigue, tiredness Lack of willpower Impotence, infertility, lack of sexual desire Excessive urination Chilling in lower body
	Strengthens Kidney function of receiving Ki	Chronic Asthma
	Strengthens Lower Back	Chronic lower backache
	Benefits Bones and Marrow	Arthritic bone deformities Dizziness Poor memory Weak legs
	Benefits Ears and Eyes	Tinnitus, deafness Chronic eye disorders, poor vision, dry eyes
	Nourishes Blood	Anaemia Menstrual syndromes: absence of menses, irregular menstruation, menstrual pain
	Resolves Dampness	Fullness of Bladder, with feeling of distension Urinary stones

IDENTIFICATION	ACTION	INDICATIONS
BL 25 Dachangshu LARGE INTESTINE'S HOLLOW 1.5 SUN lateral to the centre of the SPINE between the 4th and 5th LUMBAR VERTEBRA LARGE INTESTINE YU/SHU or BACK TRANSPORTING POINT	Promotes LI function Strengthens Lower Back	Constipation, diarrhoea, flatulence Chronic LI disease: Diverticulitis, Colitis etc. Abdominal fullness, distension Rectal prolapse Acute/chronic backache Sciatica Stiffness
BL 27 Xiaochangshu SMALL INTESTINE'S HOLLOW 1.5 SUN lateral to the centre of the SACRAL SPINE, level with the 1st SACRAL FORAMEN SMALL INTESTINE YU/SHU or BACK TRANSPORTING POINT	Promotes SI function Resolves Dampness Lower Heater	Abdominal pain, intestinal rumbling Mucus in stools Diarrhoea Cloudy and difficult urination Inflammation of Bladder (Cystitis)
BL 28 Pangguangshu BLADDER'S HOLLOW 1.5 SUN lateral to the centre of the SACRAL SPINE, level with the 2nd SACRAL FORAMEN BLADDER YU/SHU or BACK TRANSPORTING POINT	Regulates Bladder Clears Heat/Dampness Lower Heater Opens Water Passages Strengthens Lower Back	Urinary incontinence Urination with seminal discharge Urinary tract infection Blood in the urine Inflammation of Prostrate Gland Burning on urination Oedema Frequent urination Sacroiliac pain or stiffness Sciatica Coldness in lower body or pelvis Lower back or pelvic pain
BL 40 Weizhong SUPPORTING MIDDLE Mid point of the transverse crease of the POPLITEAL FOSSA located between the TENDONS of the BICEPS FEMORIS and SEMITENDINOSUS muscles SEA POINT EARTH POINT **** Use Moxibustion with caution ****	Removes Channel obstructions Resolves Dampness Cools Blood Clears Heat Eliminates Blood stasis	Acute backache/Sciatica Burning on urination Skin diseases of a heat nature i.e. Herpes Zoster Fever and delirium Varicose veins Lower leg pain

RESIDENTIAL TSUBO STUDIES

IDENTIFICATION	ACTION	INDICATIONS
BL 57 Chengshan SUPPORTING MOUNTAIN 8 SUN below BL 40, inferior to the belly of the GASTROCNEMIUS muscle on a line connecting BL 40 to the ACHILLES TENDON	Strengthens Lower Back Relaxes Tendons including Ligaments Invigorates Blood	Lower backache, Sciatica Cramping of the Gastrocnemius muscle Menstrual pain, blood in the stools Haemorrhoids, varicose veins Rectal prolapse
BL 60 Kunlun KUNLUN MOUNTAINS Between the posterior border of the LATERAL MALLEOLUS and the medial aspect of the ACHILLES TENDON, level with the vertex of the LATERAL MALLEOLUS RIVER POINT FIRE POINT **** Contraindicated in pregnancy ****	Strengthens the Lower Back Painful obstruction on Channel Disperses Int/Ext Wind Expedites Labour Clears Heat	Chronic backache presenting in deficiency pattern Shoulder, neck and occipital pain or stiffness Sciatica Ankle/heel pain Difficult labour Burning urination
BL 67 Zhiyin REACHING YIN About 0.1 SUN from the lateral corner of the 5th TOENAIL WELL POINT METAL POINT **** Contraindicated during pregnancy except as indicated ****	Eliminates Int/Ext Wind Calms Foetus Used at 8th month of pregnancy with MOXA Expedites Labour	Headaches Nasal congestion and discharge Blurred and painful eyes Breech presentation (malposition of foetus) Difficult labour

RESIDENTIAL TSUBO STUDIES

IDENTIFICATION	ACTION	INDICATIONS
KD 1 Yongquan BUBBLING SPRING In a depression on the sole when the FOOT is plantar flexed, one third the distance from a line between the base of the 2nd and 3rd TOES and the back centre of the HEEL WELL POINT WOOD POINT	Tonifies Yin Calms the Mind Clears Fire and Heat Subdues Wind	Infertility Oedema Kidney and back pain Sensation of heat in the soles of the feet Extreme fear, insomnia, severe anxiety Shock, mental illness Loss of consciousness Dizziness, epilepsy High blood pressure Headaches presenting at the top of the head
KD 3 Taixi GREAT STREAM Midway between the MEDIAL MALLEOLUS and the ACHILLES TENDON level with the vertex of the MEDIAL MALLEOLUS SOURCE POINT STREAM POINT EARTH POINT	Tonifies the Kidneys and Essence Strengthens Original Ki Regulates the Uterus Strengthens the Lower Back and Knees	Chronic tiredness Impotence Tinnitus Urinary dysfunction Kidney inflammation Lack of willpower Bone problems Infertility Irregular menstruation, absence of menstruation, excessive bleeding Chronic lower backache Knee problems
KD 7 Fuliu RETURNING CURRENT 2 SUN directly superior to KD 3 on the anterior border of the ACHILLES TENDON RIVER POINT METAL POINT	Tonifies the Kidneys mainly Kidney Yang Resolves Dampness Lower Heater Regulates Sweating Strengthens the Lower Back Kidney Zone	Cold feeling in the body Aversion to cold Sore back, weak knees Oedema Impotence Scanty or abundant clear urine Lack of willpower Oedema in the legs Irregular menstruation Urinary dysfunction Under or oversweating response Lower back and kidney pain
KD 27 Shufu CONVEYING PALACE 2 SUN lateral to CV Channel in the depression on the lower border of the CLAVICLE	Stimulates Kidney for reception of Ki Subdues ascending Ki	Asthma, Bronchitis, chest pain Asthma, cough, anxiety and restlessness

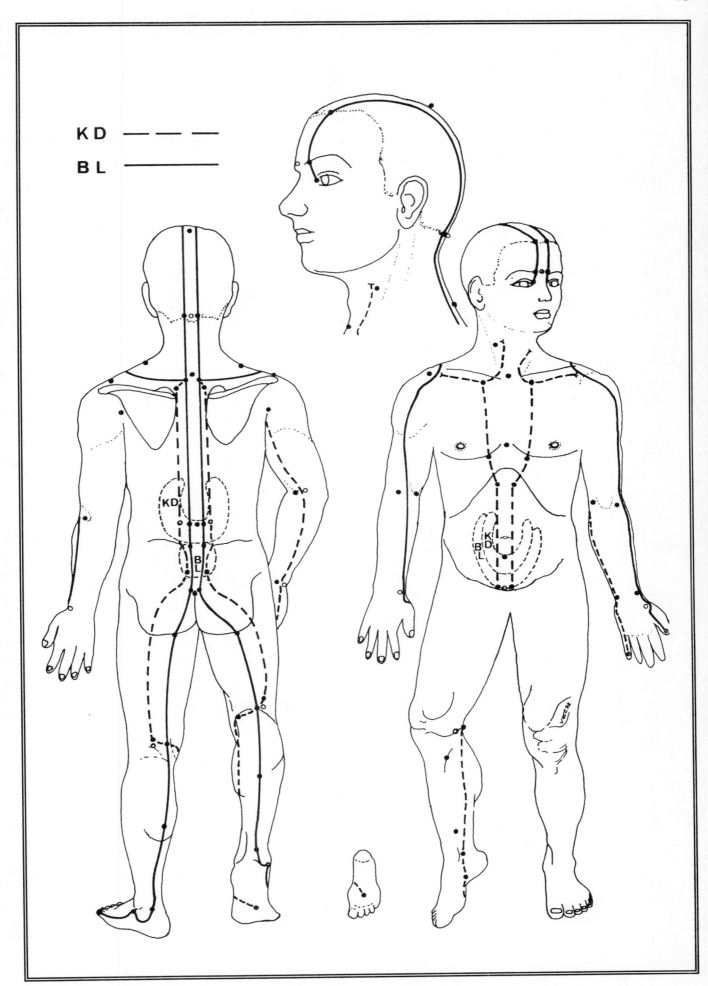

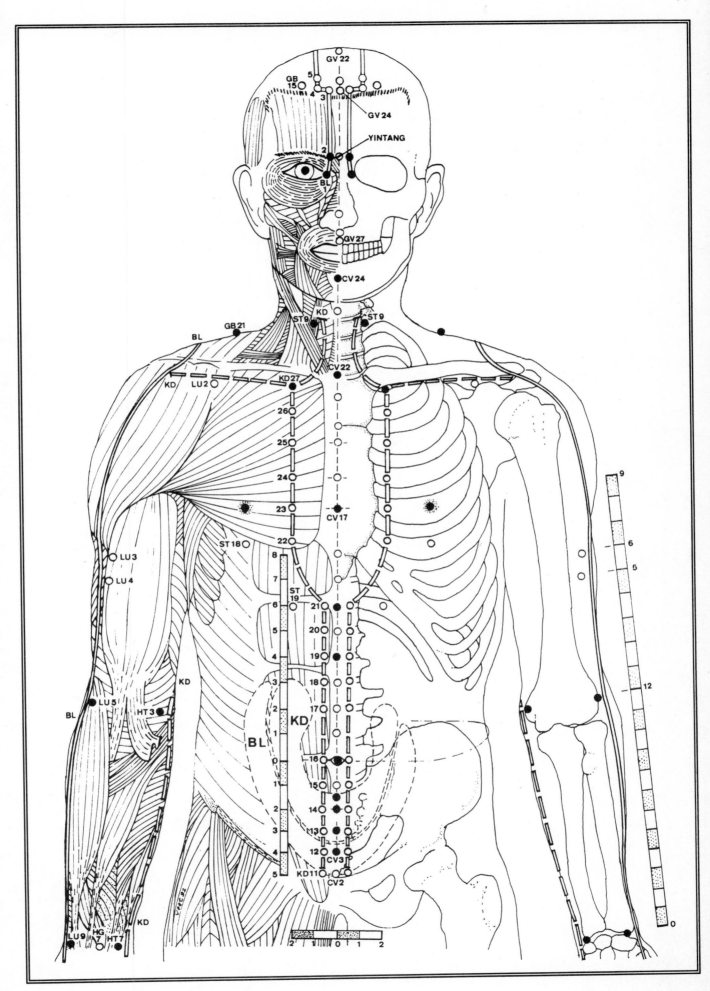

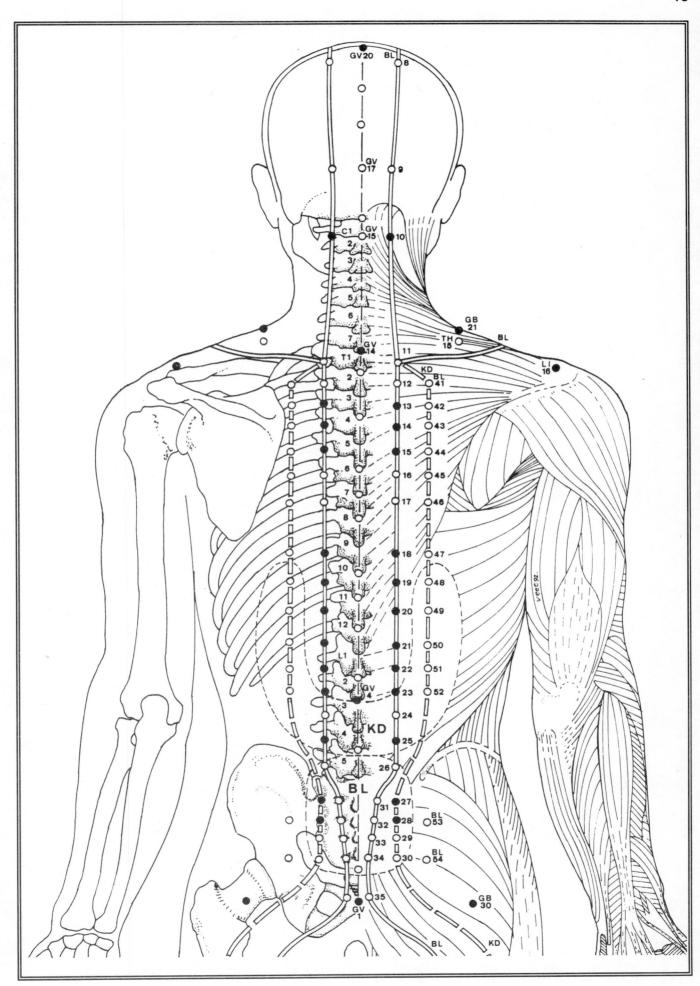

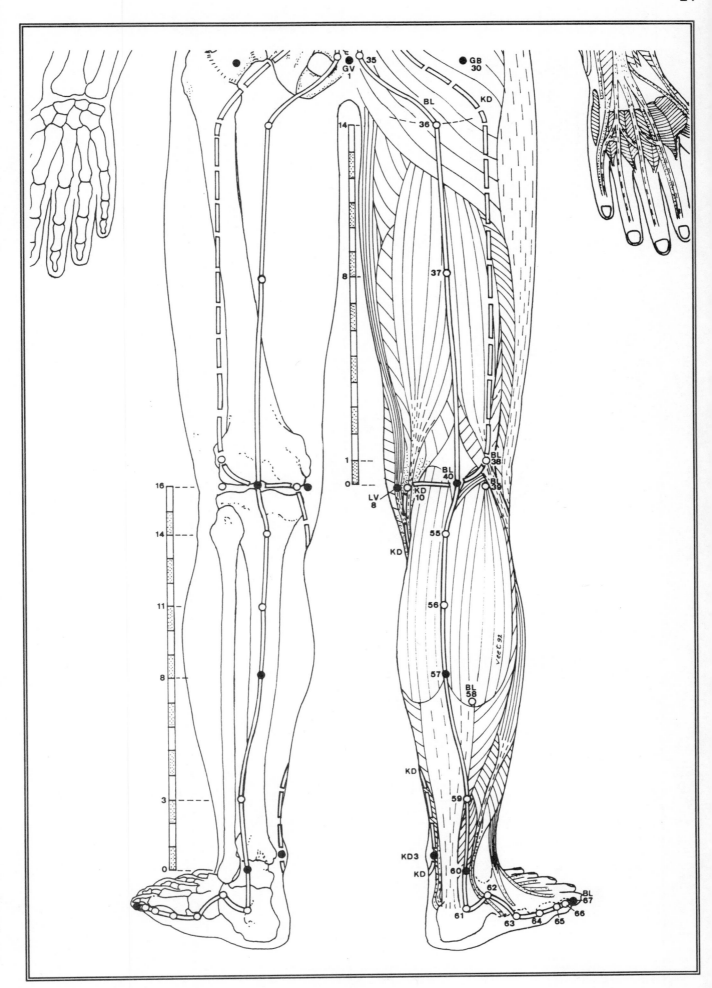

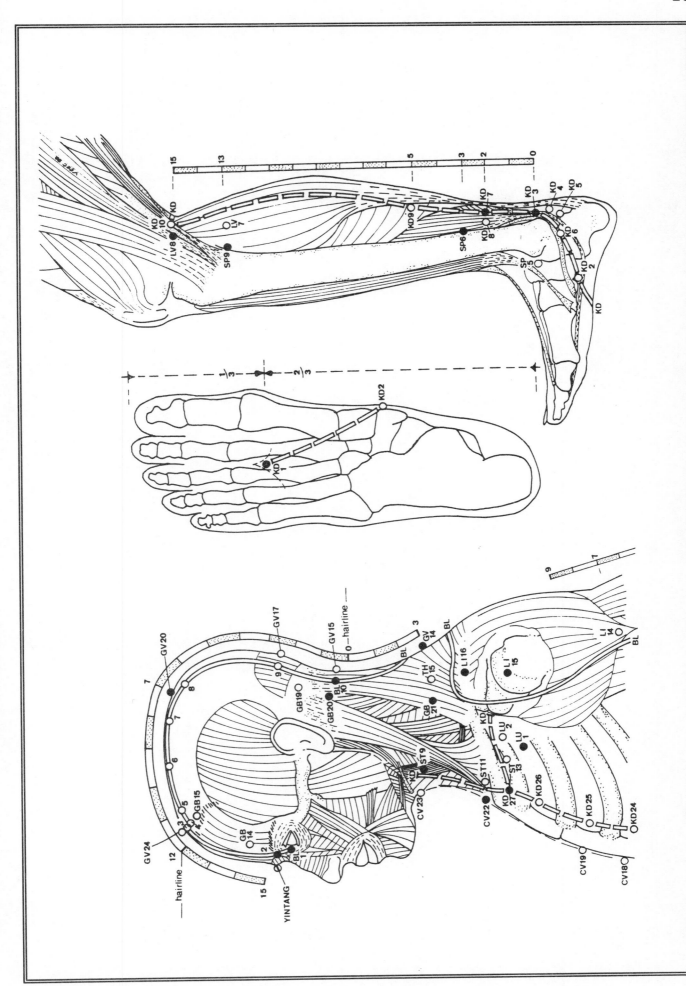

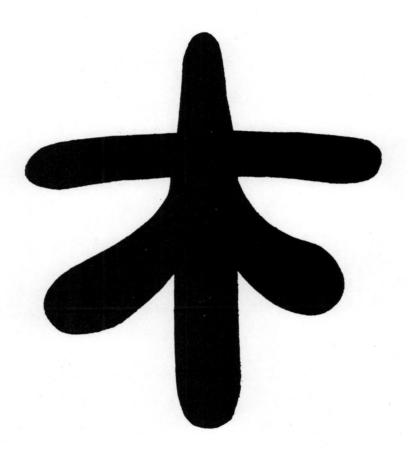

THE FIVE ELEMENT CORRESPONDENCES

FACULTY

Spiritual	Ethereal Soul
	HUN
	Planning
Genetic	Evolution
Cycle	Birth
Yin/Yang	Lesser Yang
Quality	Upward

ENVIRONMENTAL

Season	Spring
Climate	Wind
Direction	East
Part of Day	Morning,
	5am-10am
Colour	Green, Yellow

BODY

Organ	**Yin**	Liver
	Yang	Gall Bladder
Tissue		Tendons,
		Ligaments
Sense Organ		Eyes
Senses		Sight
Branch		Nails
Skin Colour		Green, Yellow
Odour		Rancid, Oily
Fluid		Tears

EMOTIONAL

Emotion	Anger
	Humour
Sound, Voice	Shouting
	Clipped
Action	Twitching

FOOD

Animal	Chicken
Fruit	Plum
Grain	Wheat, Barley
Vegetable	Sprouts
	Upward Growth
Taste	Sour

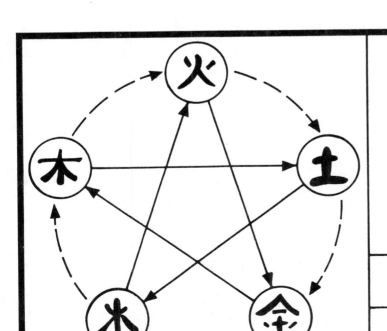

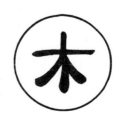

WOOD

ZEN SHIATSU MERIDIAN CORRESPONDENCES

GALL BLADDER MERIDIAN
TAN ching

FACULTY	Spiritual Input	:	HUN via Liver Meridian
	Functions via	:	Etheric Body
	Represents	:	Accomplishment
	Supplemented by	:	Decision Making
	Realised via	:	Resolving
	Dominant Zone	:	Side
	Embryological Layer	:	Mesoderm
	Meridian Nature	:	Yang
	Tuning Time	:	11pm - 1am

ANATOMY & PHYSIOLOGY	Thyroid]	Hormonal System (EGS)
	Parathyroids]	
	Gall Bladder]	Digestive System
	Pancreas]	
	Female, Male Genitalia]	Reproductive System
	Ova]	Sexual Vitality
	Spermatozoa]	
	Eyes]	Co-ordination
	Joints, Ligaments]	Musco-Skeletal System
	Tendons]	

PHYSICAL	Abdominal Distension	Lack of Sexual Response
	Biliary Pain/Gallstones	Lack of Sexual Vigour
	Bitter Taste	Jaundice, Yellow Eyes
	Blurred Vision	Joint Pain, Stiffness
	Diarrhoea	Migraine Headaches
	Difficulty Twisting	Nutritional Disorders
	Eye Problems	Pain in Flanks, Genitals
	Fatigue	Poor Digestion of Fats
	Infertility	Pyrosis (Heartburn)
	Intercostal Neuralgia	Shoulder Tension

PSYCHOLOGICAL	Agitated During Sleep	Indecisive
	Anger - Rage	Issues of Choice
	At Wits' End	Officious
	Disappointed	Overbearing
	Discriminate	Overcompetitive
	Easily Upset	Overconcentrative
	Fast Food/Life Freak	Resentment
	High Achiever	Responsibility
	Impatient	Stuckness
	Inability to Act	Tiredness after Stress

ZEN SHIATSU MERIDIAN CORRESPONDENCES

LIVER MERIDIAN
KAN ching

FACULTY		
	Spiritual Input	: HUN, Ethereal Soul
	Functions via	: Etheric Body
	Represents	: Flow of Ki
	Supplemented by	: Planning
	Realised via	: Aspiring
	Dominant Zone	: Side
	Embryological Layer	: Mesoderm
	Meridian Nature	: Yin
	Tuning Time	: 1am - 3am

ANATOMY & PHYSIOLOGY		
	Liver	] Digestive System/Nutritional] Blood Quality
	Female, Male Genitalia Fertilised Egg (Zygote)	] Hormonal System (EGS)] Reproductive System] Sexual Vitality] Reproduction/Early Development
	Eyes Joints, Ligaments Tendons	] Co-ordination] Musco-Skeletal System]
	Nails	] Integumentary System

PHYSICAL		
	Alcohol Poisoning Cracked Nails Dizziness Eye, Visual Disorders Fevers Flatulence Haemorrhoids Hypochondriac Pain Infertility Jaundice	Joint Pain, Stiffness Lack of Sexual Energy Liver Problems Migraine Headaches Nausea Poor Digestion (Fats) Sexual Organ Dysfunctions Sluggish due to Toxins — Tension in Flanks Weight Loss

PSYCHOLOGICAL		
	Anger Bad Tempered Depression Disappointment Easily Disturbed Emotionally Sensitive Irritable Lack of Patience Loud Mouthed Observer	Opinionated Overdemanding Overindulgence Perseverance Psycho-sexual Endurance Repressed Emotions Resentment Sudden Inspiration Tunnel Vision Worry over Future

FUNCTIONAL SYSTEM	MERIDIAN / ORGAN FUNCTIONS IN ORIENTAL MEDICINE	

ZANGFU	LIVER GAN	GALL BLADDER DAN
	Ensures the smooth flow of Ki Stores the Blood Controls the Sinews (Tendons & Ligaments) Opens into the Eyes Manifests in the Nails Houses the Ethereal Soul (HUN)	Stores and excretes Bile Controls judgement Controls the Sinews
IMAGE	Like an **Army General** who plans the Overall Strategy	The impartial **Officer** who makes Decisions
CHINESE GOVT POST	**GENERAL**	**LIEUTENANT**

ZEN SHIATSU	LIVER Meridian KAN ching	GALL BLADDER Meridian TAN ching
	Stores Nutrients and vital Energy **Plans distribution of Energy** **Stores and detoxifies Blood** **Cultivates resistance against Disease**	**Distribution of Nutrients to Body** **Balances Energy through Hormones, Bile secretion, Gastric Acid and Insulin** **Responds to Liver's Plans by deciding Course of Action**
BASIC	**Detoxification, Planning and Storage of Ki**	**Delivers Nutrients for Maintenance**
SPECIFIC	PLANNING	DECISION MAKING
GENERAL	DISTRIBUTION OF KI	

IDENTIFICATION	ACTION	INDICATIONS
GB 1 Tongziliao PUPILS CREVICE 0.5 SUN lateral to the OUTER CANTHUS of the EYE GB, TH, SI MEETING POINT	Clears Wind Heat Clears Fire Brightens the Eyes	Conjunctivitis Red, dry, painful eyes Migraine headaches Night/Colour blindness Dislike of light
GB 12 Wangu WHOLE BONE In the depression immediately posterior and inferior to the MASTOID process GB, BL MEETING POINT	Subdues Rising Ki Dispels Wind Exterior and Interior Calms the Mind	Posterior migraine headaches on the GB channel Earache and toothache Epilepsy Inflammation of the Middle Ear Insomnia, throat pain and stiff neck due to emotional crisis
GB 20 Fengchi WIND POOL In the hollow between the OCCIPITAL PROTRUBERANCE and the MASTOID bone, level with GV 16 and between the upper SCM muscle and TRAPEZIUS muscle	Dispels Wind Exterior and Interior Subdues Liver Yang / Fire Calms the Mind Clears the Brain Sea of Marrow	EXT. Pronounced headache, stiff neck, shoulder and back pain INT Vertigo Dizziness Occipital headaches Eye and Ear problems Insomnia, dizziness, vertigo Poor memory Hypertension
GB 21 Jianjing SHOULDER WELL At the highest point of the SHOULDER, halfway between GV 14 and the ACROMION GB, TH MEETING POINT **** Contraindicated in pregnancy ****	Relaxes Tendons including Ligaments Re-directs Ki downward Promotes Delivery Facilitates Lactation	Tender and painful neck and shoulders Cough, hiccup, difficulty inhaling, Asthma Digestive problems Retention of placenta Threatened miscarriage Post Partum haemorrhage Difficult labour Insufficient lactation Mastitis

IDENTIFICATION	ACTION	INDICATIONS
GB 24 Riyue SUN AND MOON Directly below the NIPPLE in the 7th INTERCOSTAL SPACE (between the 7th and 8th RIBS) BO or COLLECTING POINT for GALL BLADDER	Damp Heat cleared from LV/GB Promotes LV/GB function Spreads Liver Ki	Jaundice Hypochondriac pain Heavy feeling in Middle Heater Nausea, sticky yellow tongue coating Gallstones Hypochondriac pain and distension Tight chest, depression Indecision
GB 25 Jingmen CAPITAL GATE At the tip of the free end of the 12th RIB BO or COLLECTING POINT for KIDNEY	Tonifies Kidneys Yin or Yang aspects Resolves Dampness Lower Heater Expels stones	Breathing problems Painful urinary dysfunction Restless foetal disorder Oedema Hypochondriac, abdominal or lower back pain Inflammation of Kidney Urinary tract stones
GB 30 Huantiao JUMPING CIRCLE One third the distance from the GREATER TROCHANTER of the FEMUR to the SACRAL HIATUS GB, BL MEETING POINT	Tonifies Ki and Blood Removes obstructions from Channel Resolves Damp Heat Lower Heater	Whole body tiredness with stagnant feeling Hip joint and leg pain Sciatica Rheumatism Itchy anus or groin Vaginal discharge Urethritis Lower back or groin pain
GB 34 Yanglingquan YANG MOUND SPRING In the hollow anterior and inferior to the head of the FIBULA SEA POINT EARTH POINT GATHERING POINT for SINEWS, TENDONS AND LIGAMENTS	Smooths Liver Ki Subdues rebellious Ki Resolves Damp Heat Relaxes Tendons including Ligaments	Hypochondriac pain Gallstones Nausea and vomiting Hepatitis Knee pain, oedema, sciatica, rheumatism, muscle atrophy Cramps and spasms **Woody** like tight musculature

IDENTIFICATION	ACTION	INDICATIONS
GB 40 Qiuxu MOUND RUINS Anterior and inferior to the LATERAL MALLEOLUS in the hollow on the lateral side of the TENDON of the EXTENSOR DIGITORUM LONGUS muscle SOURCE POINT	Smooths Liver Ki, harmonises LV/GB Removes obstructions from Channel	Gallstones Hypochondriac pain, distension with sighing Indecision Pain in neck, side, hip, knee and ankle Weak joints with swelling inc. foot
GB 44 Zuqiaoyin FOOT YIN CAVITY About 0.1 SUN from the lateral corner of the 4th TOENAIL WELL POINT METAL POINT	Subdues Liver Yang Soothes Eyes Calms the Mind	Migraine headaches Obstruction of throat Red, painful eyes Insomnia Agitation

IDENTIFICATION	ACTION	INDICATIONS
LV 1 Dadun BIG THICK At the lateral corner of the big TOENAIL WELL POINT WOOD POINT	Resolves Damp Heat Lower Heater zone Contains the Blood Spreads Liver Ki	Genital itching, swelling and pain Urinary infection and incontinence Uterine bleeding or blood in urine or stool Irregular menstruation Distension of hypogastrium Urinary pain
LV 3 Taichong GREAT RUSHING Between the 1st and 2nd TOES 2 SUN proximal to the margin of the web SOURCE POINT STREAM POINT EARTH POINT	Subdues Liver Yang Calms the Mind Smooths Liver Ki Expels Interior Wind	Migraines, headaches with dizziness Rebellious Ki Stress, irritability and frustration Repressed anger Premenstrual tension Irregular menstruation Calms spasms and cramping of the muscles
LV 4 Zhongfeng MIDDLE BARRIER On the medial side of the TENDON of the TIBIALIS ANTERIOR muscle, level with the vertex of the MEDIAL MALLEOLUS RIVER POINT METAL POINT	Smooths Liver Ki Lower Heater zone Painful obstruction syndrome	Hernial disorders Distension of hypogastrium due to stagnant Liver Ki Urinary retention Impotence Pain and swelling of the ankle
LV 8 Ququan CURVED SPRING With the KNEE flexed, in the depression of the transverse crease between the upper border of the MEDIAL EPICONDYLE of the FEMUR and the TENDON of the SEMI MEMBRANOSUS muscle SEA POINT WATER POINT	Resolves Dampness Hot or Cold Lower Heater zone Nourishes Blood Relaxes Tendons	Urinary retention Cloudy urine Burning urination Vaginal discharge Genital itching Irregular menstruation Impotence Arthritic pain Stiffness and/or swelling at the medial aspect of the thigh

IDENTIFICATION	ACTION	INDICATIONS
LV 13 Zhangmen ORDER GATE At the anterior end of the 11th RIB BO or COLLECTING POINT for SPLEEN GATHERING POINT for the 5 YIN ORGANS	Smooths Liver Ki Relieves retention of food	LV/SP disharmony Spleen Ki not ascending Loose stools Abdominal distension Stomach Ki not descending Retention of food Belching Epigastric fullness
LV 14 Qimen CYCLIC GATE On the mammillary line directly below the NIPPLE in the 6th INTERCOSTAL SPACE (between the 6th and 7th RIBS) BO or COLLECTING POINT for LIVER	Smooths Liver Ki Cools the Blood	LV/ST disharmony Stomach Ki not descending Belching Nausea, vomiting Hypochondriac pain and distension Depression Full and tight constricted chest Difficult breathing Liver fog .. can't plan Skin rashes Inflammation of the Gall Bladder and the Pancreas

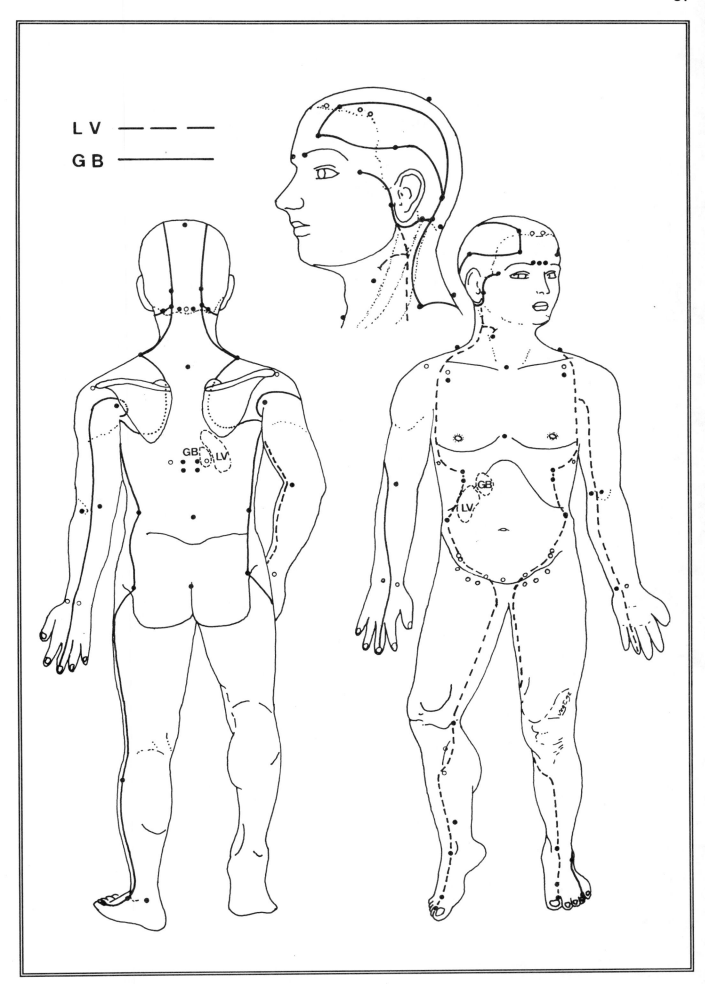

LV — — —
GB ——————

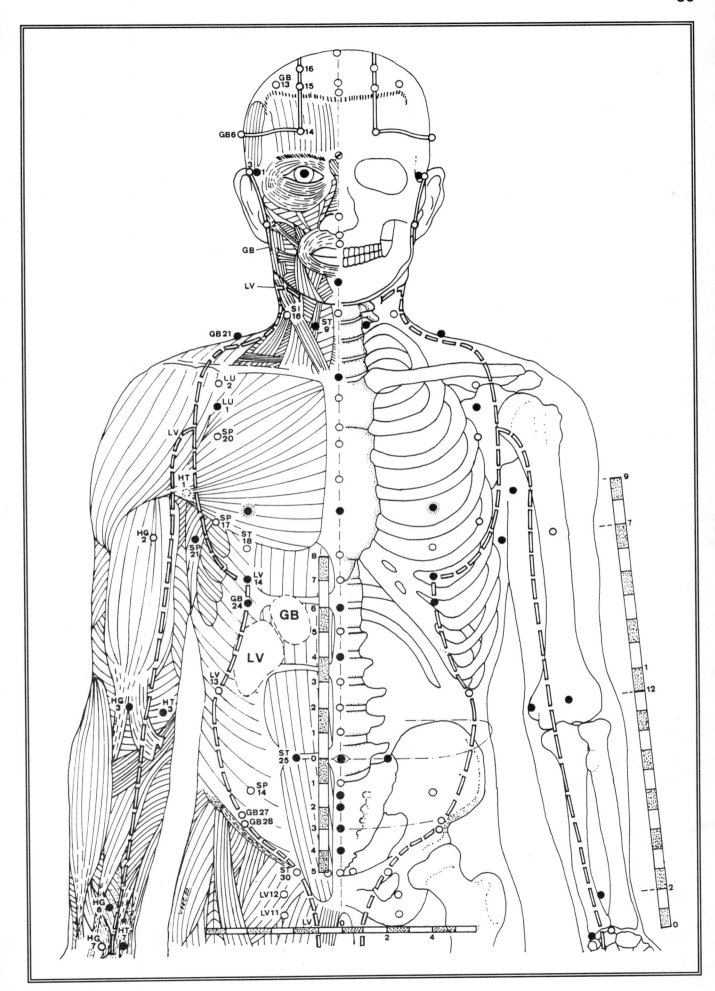

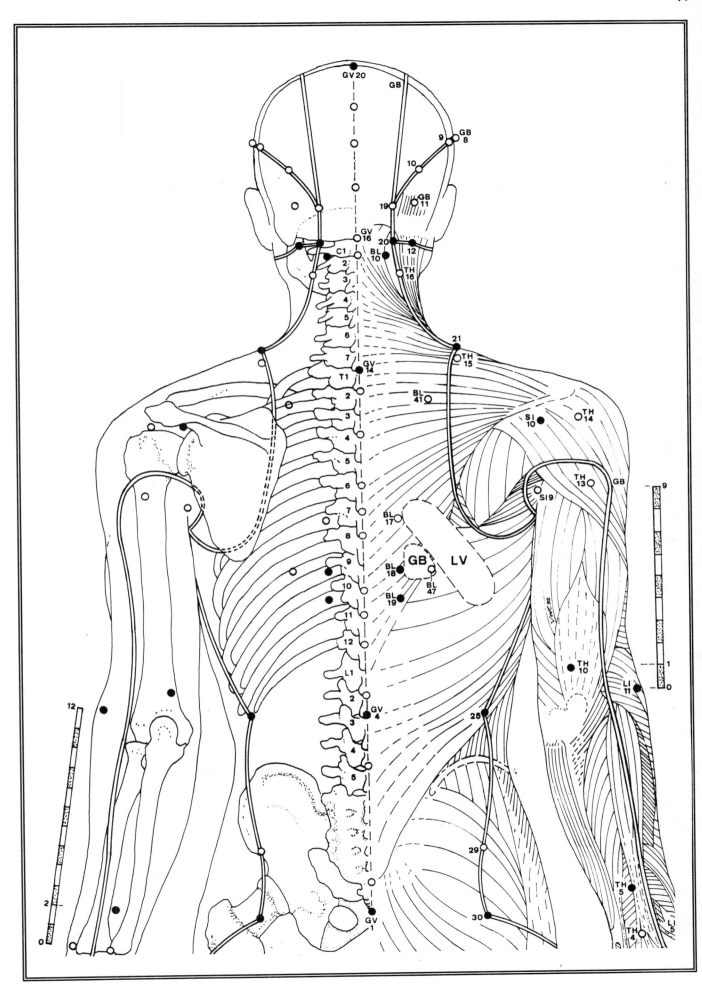

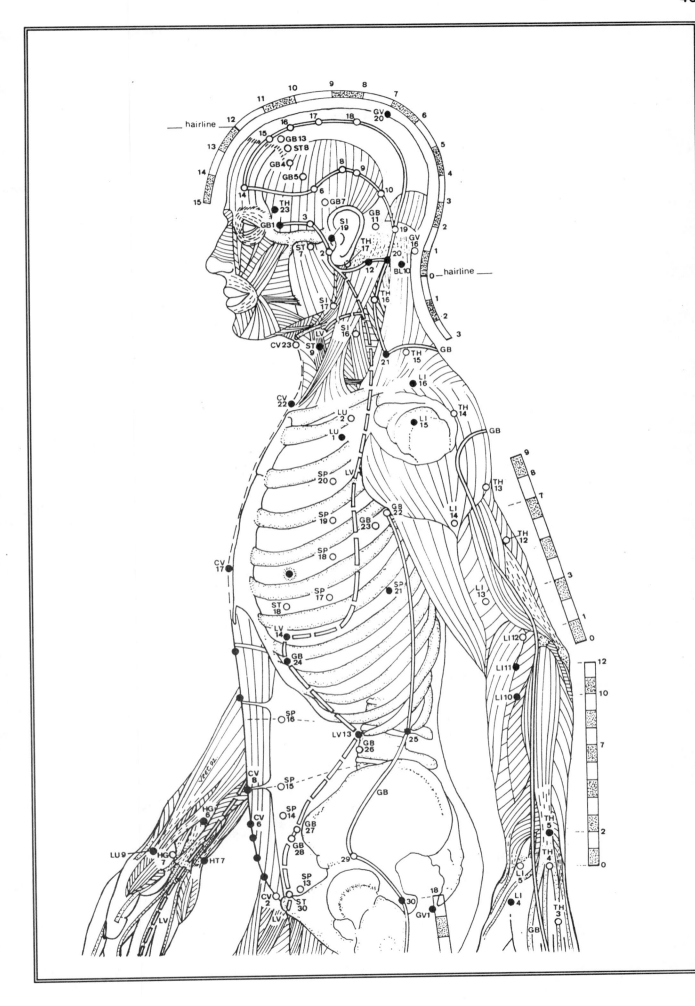

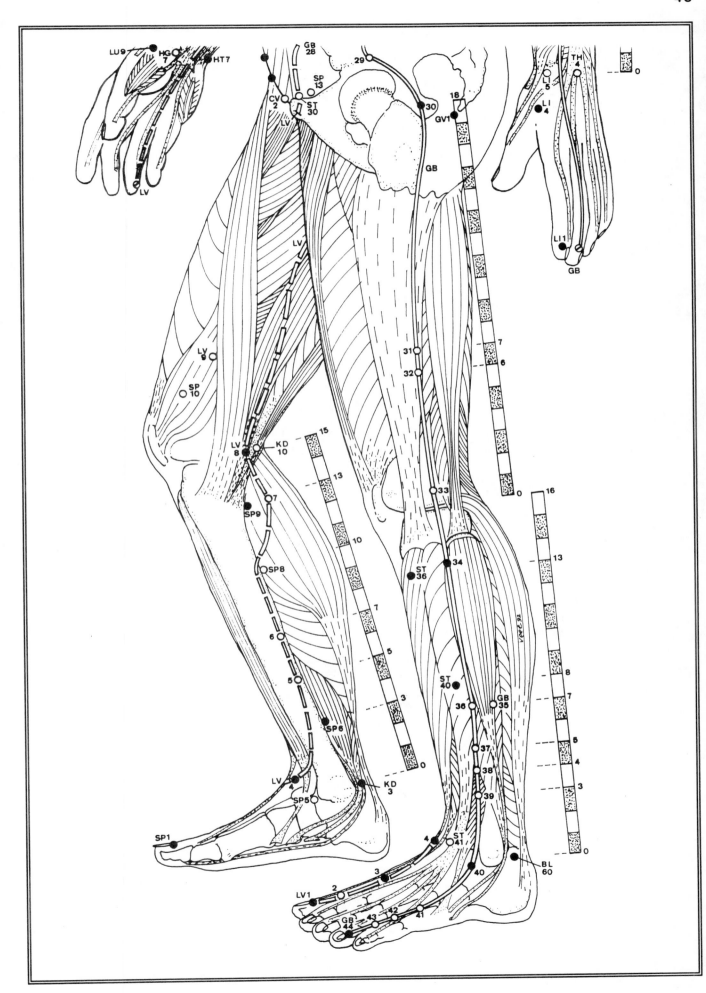

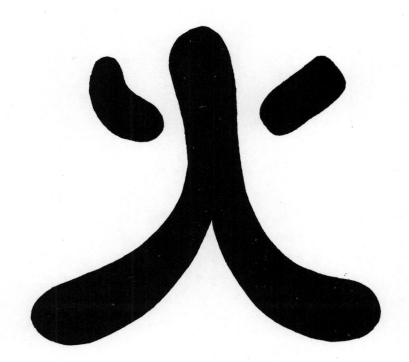

THE FIVE ELEMENT CORRESPONDENCES

FACULTY

Spiritual	Mind SHEN
	Consciousness
Genetic	Realisation
Cycle	Growth
Yin/Yang	Utmost Yang
Quality	Radiating

ENVIRONMENTAL

Season	Summer
Climate	Hot
Direction	South
Part of Day	Noon, 10am-3pm
Colour	Red

BODY

Organ	**Yin**	Heart
		Heart Governor
	Yang	Small Intestine
		Triple Heater
Tissue		Blood Vessels
Sense Organ		Tongue
Senses		Speech
Branch		Facial Colour
Skin Colour		Red, Purple
Odour		Burning
Fluid		Sweat

EMOTIONAL

Emotion	Hysteria
	Joy
Sound, Voice	Laughing
	Talkative
Action	Itching

FOOD

Animal	Sheep, Lamb
Fruit	Apricot
Grain	Corn
Vegetable	Lettuce, Enlarged
	& Leafy Greens
Taste	Bitter Hot

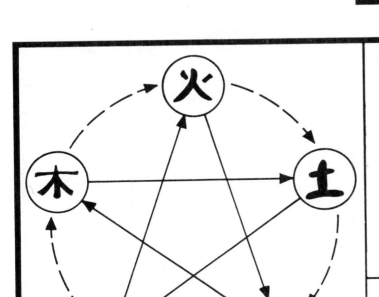

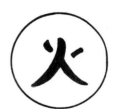

FIRE

ZEN SHIATSU MERIDIAN CORRESPONDENCES

HEART MERIDIAN
HSIN ching

FACULTY	Spiritual Input	: SHEN, Mind
	Functions via	: Consciousness
	Represents	: Awareness
	Supplemented by	: Emotional Centre
	Realised via	: Guiding
	Dominant Zone	: Inside
	Embryological Layer	: Endoderm
	Meridian Nature	: Yin
	Tuning Time	: 11am - 1pm

ANATOMY & PHYSIOLOGY	Brain	] Central Nervous System
	Spinal Cord	] (CNS)
	Eyes	] Senso-Physical Initiative
	Tongue	] Speech
	Thymus Gland	] Immune System
		] 'T' Cells Lymphocytes
	Heart	] Circulatory System
	Sinoatrial Node	] Blood Circulation
	Atrioventricular Node	]

PHYSICAL	Angina Pectoris	Myocardial Infarction
	Asthma	Oedema
	Blood Pressure Problems	Palmar Sweats
	Cardiac Arrhythmias	Palpitations
	Chest Stiffness	Poor Circulation
	Corner of Eyes - Red	Red Complexion
	Endocarditis	Rheumatic Fever
	Epigastric Tightness	Speech Problems
	Excessive Sweating	Swallowing Difficulties
	Fatigue after Exertion	Tongue Stiffness

PSYCHOLOGICAL	Adaptory Issues	Manipulative
	Anxiety	Memory Problems
	Emotional Tiredness	Nervousness
	Emotional Trauma	Neurotic
	Erratic Behaviour	Perpetual Fatigue
	Excessive Laughter	Restlessness
	Hand Tension	Stammering
	Hysteria	Talkative
	Lack of Compassion	Thirst
	Low Spirit	Worry

ZEN SHIATSU MERIDIAN CORRESPONDENCES

SMALL INTESTINE MERIDIAN
HSIAO CHANG ching

FACULTY		
	Spiritual Input	: SHEN via Heart Meridian
	Functions via	: Consciousness
	Represents	: Absorption
	Supplemented by	: Assimilation
	Realised via	: Experiencing
	Dominant Zone	: Inside
	Embryological Layer	: Endoderm
	Meridian Nature	: Yang
	Tuning Time	: 1pm - 3pm

ANATOMY & PHYSIOLOGY		
	Brain]	Cerebrospinal Fluid (CSF)
	Spinal Cord]	
	Small Intestine (Ileum)]	**Digestive System**
	]	**Blood Quality**
	Ovaries]	**Hormonal System**
	]	**Reproductive System**

PHYSICAL		
	Anaemia	**Hearing Disorders**
	Appendicitis	Hip Pain, Sciatica
	Blood Disorders	Lordosis & Lumbar Pain
	Borborygmi	Malabsorption
	Chilly Extremities	Menstrual Problems
	Constipation	Migraine Headaches
	Diarrhoea	Neck & Back Stiffness
	Ear & Jaw Pain	Physical Injury, Trauma
	Enteritis & Fever	Reproductive Problems
	Fatigued Easily	Toothache

PSYCHOLOGICAL		
	Acceptance	Overdetermination
	Concentration	Over Focused
	Confidence Issues	Patience
	Discriminate Nature	Restless
	Emotional Trauma	Righteous
	Experimentation	Selfish
	Indecisive	Shock
	Judgemental	Sorrowful
	Lack of Reality	Suppression of Feelings
	Obsession with Small Details	Wanting It All

ZEN SHIATSU MERIDIAN CORRESPONDENCES

HEART GOVERNOR MERIDIAN
HSIN PAO ching

FACULTY

Spiritual Input	:	SHEN via Heart Meridian
Functions via	:	Consciousness
Represents	:	Interpretation
Supplemented by	:	Vascular Response
Realised via	:	Communicating
Dominant Zone	:	Surface
Embryological Layer	:	Ectoderm
Meridian Nature	:	Yin
Tuning Time	:	7pm - 9pm

ANATOMY & PHYSIOLOGY

Meninges]
Pericardium] Central Nervous System
Heart] (CNS)
Aorta] Systemic & Pulmonary
Major Arteries/Veins] Circulation

Thoracic & Right Lymphatic
Ducts] Lymphatic System

PHYSICAL

Angina Pectoris	Palpitations
Blood Pressure Disorders	Pins & Needles
Chest Pain, Stiffness	Poor Working Posture
Circulatory Disorders	Pulse Irregularities
Cold Extremities	Pyloric Pain, Stiffness
Head Haziness	Pyrosis (Heartburn)
Heart Disorders	Throat Inflammation/Fever
Insomnia	Tiredness on Exertion
Meningitis	Tonsillitis
Oedema	Wheezing

PSYCHOLOGICAL

Absent Minded	Lack of Reality
Breathing Difficulties	Negotiative
Can't Explain Things	Obsessed with Moving Things
Disturbed Sleep	Oppressive Feeling in Chest
Easily Startled	Overactive
Emotional Trauma	Overfocused on Work
Excessive Dreaming	Relationship Issues
Hypersensitive	Restlessness
Inability to Relax	Social Nervousness
Joyfulness	Stability Issues

ZEN SHIATSU MERIDIAN CORRESPONDENCES

TRIPLE HEATER MERIDIAN
SANCHIAO ching

FACULTY		
	Spiritual Input	: SHEN via Heart Meridian
	Functions via	: Consciousness
	Represents	: Maintenance
	Supplemented by	: Lymphatic Response
	Realised via	: Guarding
	Dominant Zone	: Surface
	Embryological Layer	: Ectoderm
	Meridian Nature	: Yang
	Tuning Time	: 9pm - 11pm

ANATOMY & PHYSIOLOGY		
	Meninges	] Central Nervous System (CNS)
	Lymph Nodes, Tissues & Vessels	] Lymphatic System
	Spleen	] Immune Response
	Mucous, Serous Membranes	] Lymphocytes, Phagocytosis
	Thyroid	] Thermo Regulatory Metabolism
	Skin	] Connective Tissue
	Fascia	] Peripheral Circulation
	Capillaries	]
	Cystic, Gastric, Mesenteric, Splenic Veins	] Portal Circulation

PHYSICAL		
	Allergies	Neck Pain
	Colds, Sneezing	Oedema
	Dizziness	Poor Circulation-Extremities
	Eczema, Urticaria	Psoriasis
	Excess Mucous Secretion	Sensitive Skin
	Eye, Throat Infections	Sensitive to Temperature Changes
	Headaches	Sneezing
	Immune Deficiency	Swollen Lymph Glands/Nodes
	Meningitis	Tight Chest & Abdomen
	Nasal Problems	Tonsillitis

PSYCHOLOGICAL		
	Armouring (Body Mind)	Over Mothered
	Awkward Stance	Overly Cautious
	Burdened	Pretentious
	Confidence Issues	Protective Attitude
	Disorganised	Relationship Problems
	Focused on Tidiness	Sensitive to Change
	Hardness	Social Problems
	Hides behind Others	Stunned
	Hypersensitive	Trauma
	Overactive	Unadventurous

FUNCTIONAL SYSTEM	MERIDIAN / ORGAN FUNCTIONS IN ORIENTAL MEDICINE	

ZANGFU	HEART XIN	SMALL INTESTINE XIAO CHANG
	Governs Blood (XUE) Controls the Blood Vessels (XUEMAI) Manifests in the Complexion Opens into the Tongue Controls Sweat Houses the Mind (SHEN)	Separates Pure from Impure Foods and Fluids for Absorption and Transformation
IMAGE	The **Monarch** who rules through insight and understanding	The **Official** in charge of screening substances for nourishment and transformation
CHINESE GOVT POST	**KING**	**KINGS SECRETARY**

ZEN SHIATSU	HEART Meridian HSIN ching	SMALL INTESTINE Meridian HSIAO CHANG ching
	Centre of Emotional response/ reaction Governs Central Nervous Systems (CNS) Controls Blood Circulation and assists Immune System Represents Awareness and Compassion	Digests and assimilates Food from the Jejunum through the Ileum to the Ileocaecal Valve Produces Blood Maintains Composure through Shock Mechanism (Blood, CSF, Ovaries, Testes)
BASIC	**Environmental Interpretation for Body Mind**	**Conversion and Integration of Nurturing Substances**
SPECIFIC	EMOTIONAL CENTRE	ASSIMILATION
GENERAL	CONTROL	

FUNCTIONAL SYSTEM	MERIDIAN / ORGAN FUNCTIONS IN ORIENTAL MEDICINE	

ZANGFU	HEART GOVERNOR X I N B A O	TRIPLE HEATER S A N J I A O
	Protects the Heart (XIN) Governs Blood (XUE) Controls the Blood Vessels (XUEMAI) Guides Joy and Pleasure	Regulates JINYE Metabolism
IMAGE	The **Palace Official** from whom pleasure and mirth are derived	The **Official** in charge of the Waterworks
CHINESE GOVT POST	**KINGS AMBASSADOR**	**WATER ENGINEER**

ZEN SHIATSU	HEART GOVERNOR Meridian H S I N P A O ching	TRIPLE HEATER Meridian S A N C H I A O ching
	Governs the Vascular System and central Lymphatic Ducts Assists Heart control central circulation Protects and assists Heart in emotional response/reaction	Governs the Lymphatic System, Portal and Peripheral Circulation and Immune System Regulates the Distribution of Nutrients from the Mesentery to the Extremities Produces and regulates Heat via Metabolism Regulates Connective Tissue and Fascia
BASIC	**Circulates Nutrients and vital Information for Life Process**	**Directs Nutrients and Instructions for Defence Mechanisms**
SPECIFIC	STABILISES BODY VIA VASCULAR RESPONSE	MAINTAINS BODY VIA LYMPHATIC RESPONSE
GENERAL	PROTECTION	

RESIDENTIAL TSUBO STUDIES

IDENTIFICATION	ACTION	INDICATIONS
HT 1 Jiquan SUPREME SPRING At the centre of the ARMPIT on the medial side of the AXILLARY ARTERY	Nourishes Heart Yin Clears Empty Fire Relaxes Chest and Shoulder	Dry mouth, night sweating, mental restlessness and insomnia Chest and cardiac pain Shoulder problems and arm pain
HT 3 Shaohai LESSER YIN SEA At the medial end of the transverse CUBITAL crease in the depression anterior to the MEDIAL EPICONDYLE of the HUMERUS SEA POINT WATER POINT	Clears Heat Calms the Mind Removes obstructions from Channel	Insomnia, epilepsy, dizziness, depression, restlessness and forgetfulness Arm, chest and elbow pain
HT 7 Shenmen SPIRIT'S GATE On the transverse WRIST crease on the RADIAL side of the FLEXOR CARPI ULNARIS muscle SOURCE POINT STREAM POINT EARTH POINT	Nourishes Heart Blood Calms the Mind	Asthmatic wheezing Hypertension Chest pain with palpitations, insomnia, poor memory, pale tongue and dizziness
HT 9 Shaochong LESSER YIN RUSHING About 0.1 SUN from the RADIAL corner of the 5th FINGERNAIL WELL POINT WOOD POINT	Clears Heat Opens Heart orifices Restores consciousness	Anxiety, hysteria, hypomania, chest pain due to emotional stress Coma, sudden loss of consciousness

RESIDENTIAL TSUBO STUDIES

IDENTIFICATION	ACTION	INDICATIONS
SI 1 Shaoze LESSER MARSH About 0.1 SUN from the ULNAR corner of the 5th FINGERNAIL WELL POINT METAL POINT	Expels Wind-Heat (Exterior invasion)	Stiff neck, headache, acute tonsillitis
	Opens Orifices	Deafness, tinnitus, and tongue stiffness
	Removes Channel obstructions	Acute or chronic neck problems
	Promotes Lactation	Mastitis and insufficient lactation
SI 3 Houxi BACK STREAM At the end of the transverse crease proximal to the 5th METACARPO-PHALANGEAL joint on the ULNAR side when the HAND is half clenched STREAM POINT WOOD POINT OPENING POINT OF GV	Eliminates Int. Wind from Governing Vessel	Convulsions, tremors, epilepsy, stiff neck, dizziness and headache
	Expels Ext. Wind	Stiff neck, occipital headache, spinal aches and chills and fever
	Resolves Dampness	Jaundice and heaviness in the chest
	Benefits Sinews	Acute upper back pain along SI, BL & GV channels
	Clears the Mind	Tendency for detailed thinking resulting in indecisiveness
SI 8 Xiaohai SMALL INTESTINE SEA With the ELBOW flexed, in the posterior aspect of the CUBITAL joint, in the FOSSA between the ULNAR OLECRANON and the MEDIAL EPICONDYLE of the HUMERUS SEA POINT EARTH POINT	Resolves Damp Heat	Acute swelling of the neck glands
	Removes Channel obstructions	Elbow and neck pain
	Calms the Mind	Anxiety
SI 9 Jianzhen UPRIGHT SHOULDER With the ARM at the side, located 1 SUN superior to the posterior end of the AXILLARY fold	Removes Channel obstructions	Pain, stiffness in shoulder, scapula or arm

IDENTIFICATION	ACTION	INDICATIONS
SI 10 Naoshu SCAPULA'S HOLLOW With the ARM at the side, located directly superior to SI9 in the depression inferior and lateral to the SCAPULAR SPINE	Removes Channel obstructions	Frozen shoulder, pain, stiffness in shoulder, scapula or arm
SI 11 Tianzong HEAVEN'S WORSHIP 1 SUN inferior to the midpoint of the lower border of the SCAPULAR SPINE	Removes Channel obstructions Relaxes Chest	Pain, stiffness in shoulder, scapula or arm Asthma, cough
SI 19 Tinggong PALACE OF HEARING With the MOUTH slightly opened, located in the depression between the TRAGUS and the MANDIBULAR joint SI, GB, TH MEETING POINT	Benefits the Ears	Deafness, tinnitus, all ear disorders

IDENTIFICATION	ACTION	INDICATIONS
HG 1 Tianchi HEAVENLY POND 1 SUN lateral to the NIPPLE, in the 4th INTERCOSTAL SPACE HG, LV MEETING POINT	Clears stagnant Liver Ki	Chest fullness Hypochondriac pain (under ribs)
HG 3 Quze CURVED MARSH With the ELBOW flexed, on the transverse CUBITAL crease, on the ULNAR side of the TENDON of the BICEPS BRACHII muscle SEA POINT WATER POINT	Clears Heat Cools Blood Calms the Mind	Heatstroke Inflammation of Stomach or Intestines Skin eruptions Fever Severe anxiety, palpitations
HG 6 Neiguan INNER GATE 2 SUN proximal to the WRIST crease between the TENDONS of the PALMARIS LONGUS and FLEXOR CARPI RADIALIS muscles CONNECTING POINT	Opens the Chest Subdues rebellious Stomach Ki Calms the Mind	All chest problems Stagnant type chest pain Nausea and vomiting Travel sickness Stomach pain Heartburn, hiccup and belching Irritability and anxiety Pre-menstrual pain, depression and restlessness
HG 8 Laogong LABOUR PALACE On the palm, on the RADIAL side of the 3rd METACARPAL bone, proximal to the METACARPO PHALANGEAL joint SPRING POINT FIRE POINT	Clears Heart Fire Calms the Mind	Mental symptoms High fever and delirium Excessive thirst Tongue ulcers Restlessness Emotional pain
HG 9 Zhongchong MIDDLE RUSHING On the middle of the tip of the middle FINGER WELL POINT WOOD POINT	Clears Heat Expels Wind Restores consciousness	Mental symptoms Heatstroke Chest or gastric pain Loss of consciousness

IDENTIFICATION	ACTION	INDICATIONS
TH 1 Guanchong GATE'S RUSHING About 0.1 SUN from the lateral corner of the 4th FINGERNAIL WELL POINT METAL POINT	Clears Heat Expels Wind Restores consciousness Removes Channel obstructions	Fever, sore throat or earache Loss of consciousness Painful and stiff shoulder joint
TH 5 Waiguan OUTER GATE 2 SUN above the DORSAL WRIST crease between the RADIUS and the ULNA CONNECTING POINT	Expels External Wind Heat Removes Channel obstructions Benefits the Ear Subdues Liver Yang	Fever, sore throat, slight sweating, aversion to cold Pain in the arm, shoulder, neck and hand Ear infection from Ext. Wind Heat Tinnitus or deafness from Liver Fire or Yang rising Migraine headaches on temples
TH 10 Tianjing HEAVENLY WELL 1 SUN superior to the OLECRANON in the depression made by flexing the ELBOW SEA POINT EARTH POINT	Removes Channel obstructions Resolves Dampness	Channel pain Painful elbow with stiff tendons Swelling of glands and tonsils from External Damp Heat
TH 23 Sizhukong SILK BAMBOO HOLE On the lateral border of the ORBIT at the lateral tip of the EYEBROW **** Use Moxibustion with caution ****	Expels Wind Benefits the Eyes Stops pain	Headache at outer corner of eyebrow (with Liver pattern) Any eye problems Headache on temples, facial paralysis at outer corner of eyebrow

HT _ _ _ _

SI _____

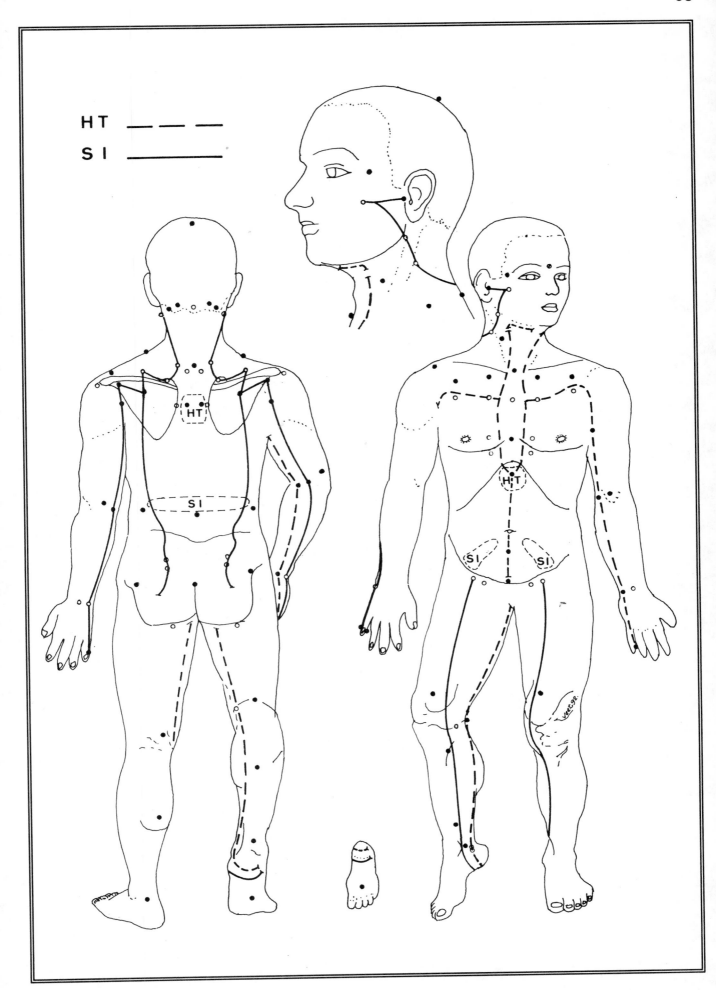

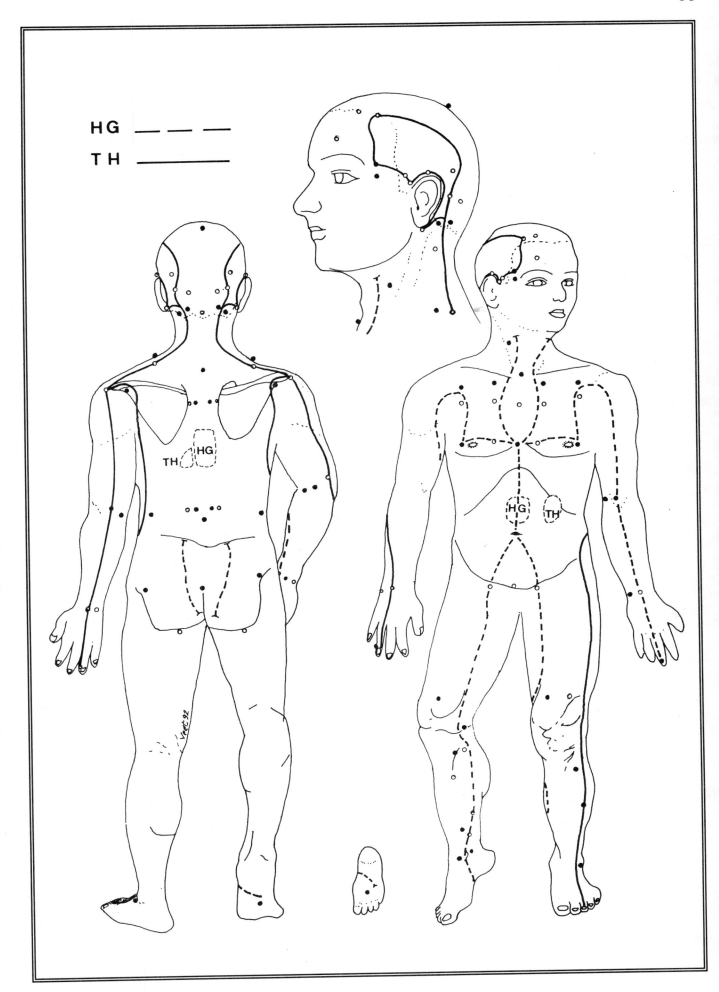

HG — — —

TH ⎯⎯⎯

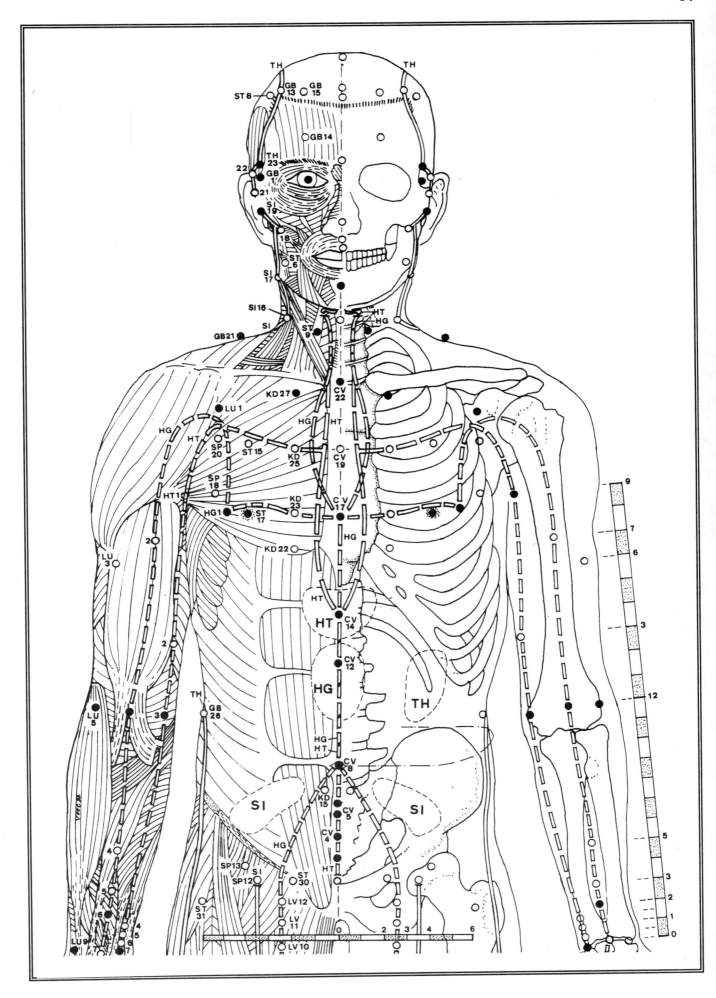

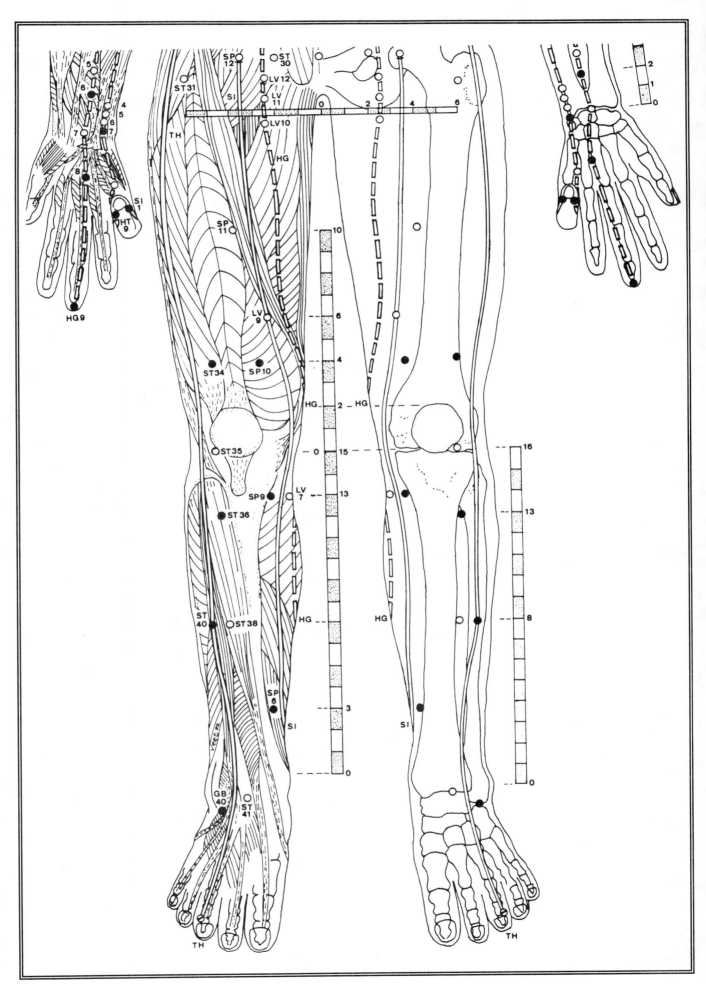

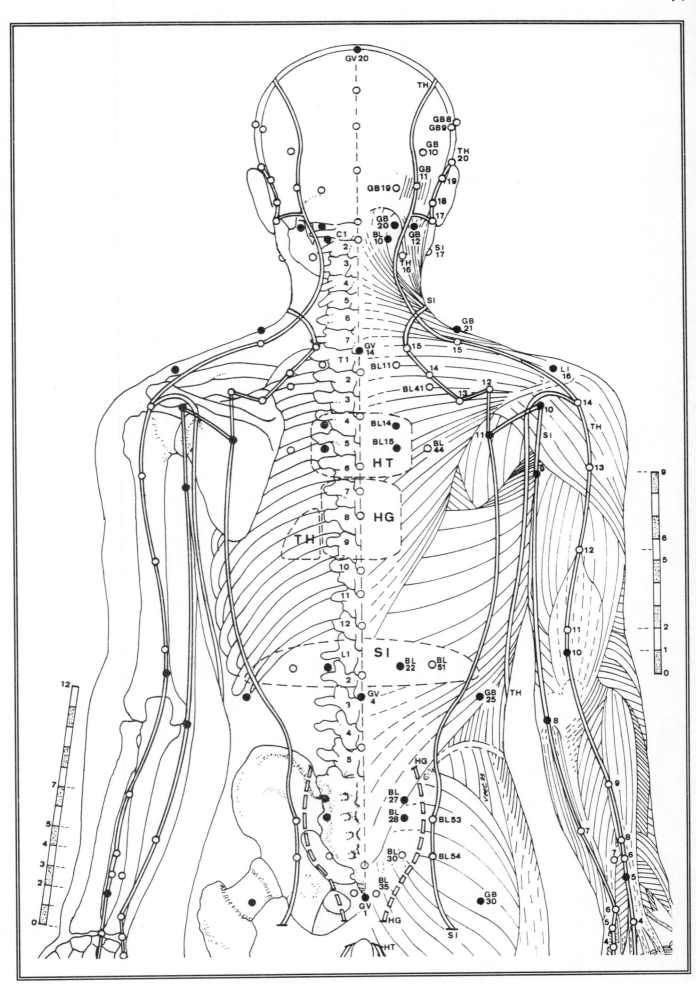

73

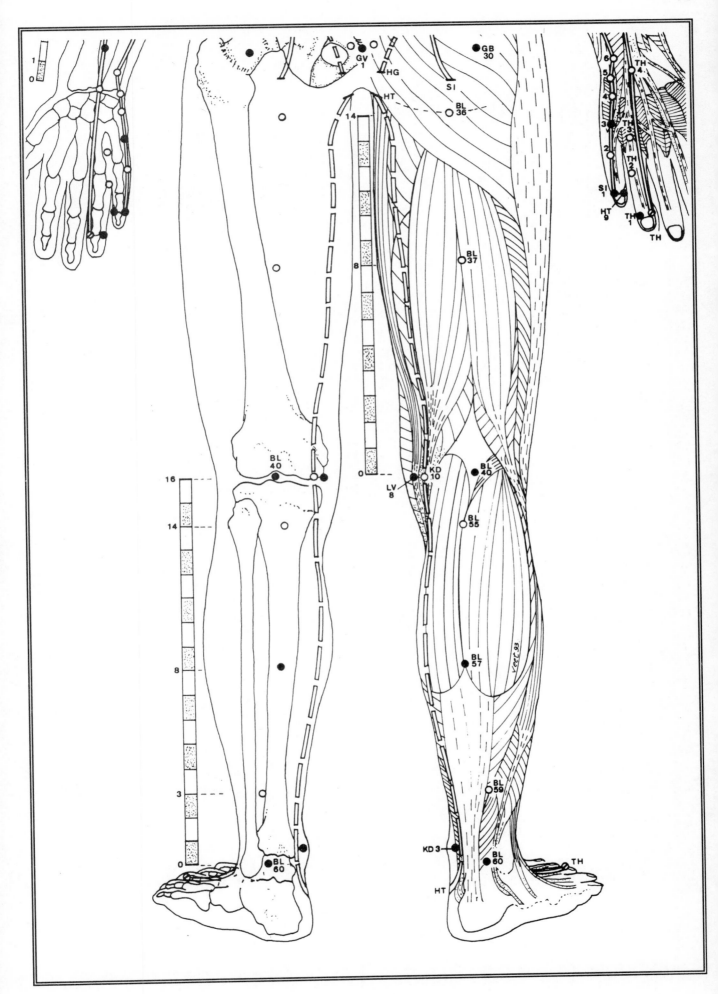

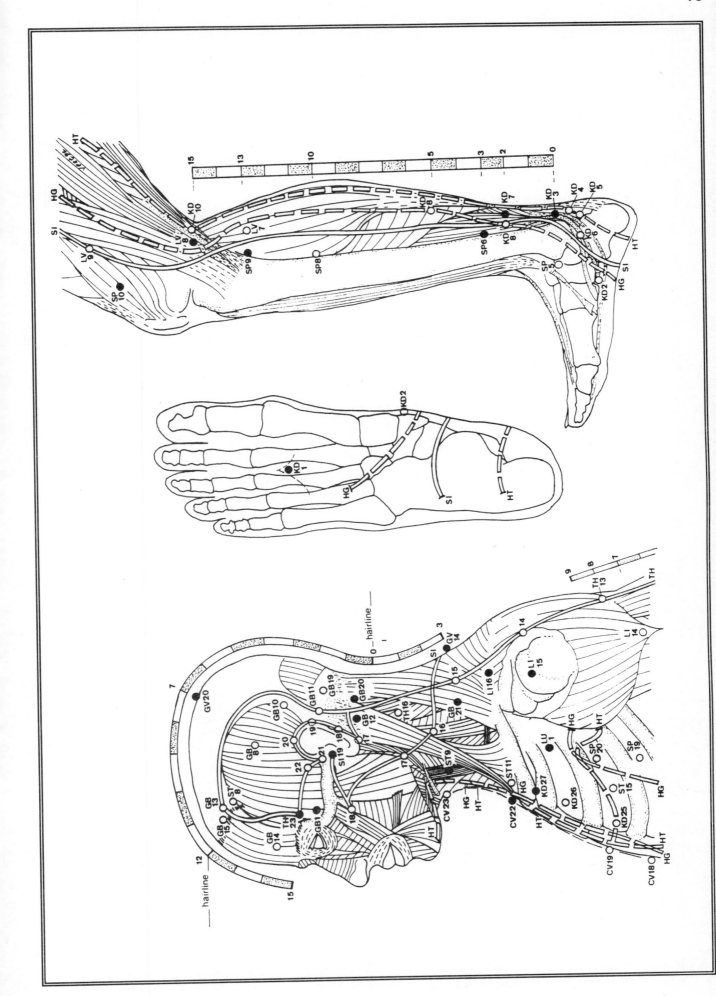

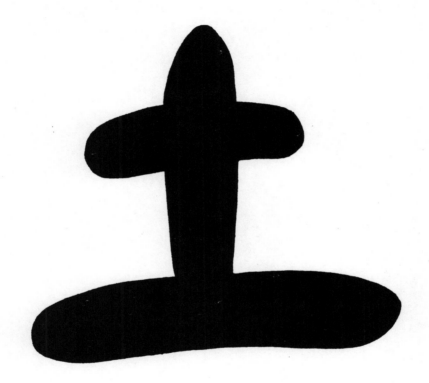

THE FIVE ELEMENT CORRESPONDENCES

FACULTY

Spiritual	Thought YI
	Intelligence
Genetic	Materialisation
Cycle	Maturity
Yin/Yang	Centre
Quality	Downward

ENVIRONMENTAL

Season	Late Summer
Climate	Humid
Direction	Centre
Part of Day	Afternoon,
	3pm-7pm
Colour	Yellow, Brown

BODY

Organ	Yin	Spleen (Pancreas)
	Yang	Stomach
Tissue		Muscle, Flesh
Sense Organ		Mouth
Senses		Taste
Branch		Lips
Skin Colour		Yellow, Brown
Odour		Fragrant
Fluid		Sticky Saliva

EMOTIONAL

Emotion	Worry
	Sympathy
Sound, Voice	Singing
	Lilting
Action	Belching

FOOD

Animal	Ox/Cow (Beef)
Fruit	Dates
Grain	Millet
Vegetable	Carrots
	Round and Sweet
Taste	Sweet

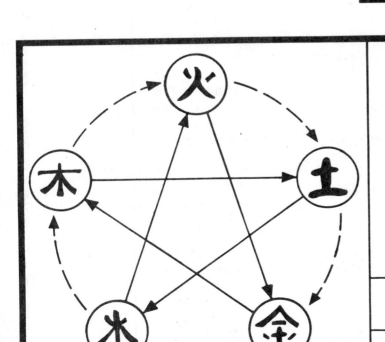

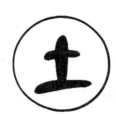

EARTH

ZEN SHIATSU MERIDIAN CORRESPONDENCES

STOMACH MERIDIAN
WEI ching

FACULTY			
	Spiritual Input	:	YI, via Spleen Meridian
	Functions via	:	Intelligence
	Represents	:	Nurturing
	Supplemented by	:	Intake of Food & Emotive Ki
	Realised via	:	Fulfilling
	Dominant Zone	:	Front
	Embryological Layer	:	Mesoderm
	Meridian Nature	:	Yang
	Tuning Time	:	7am - 9am

ANATOMY & PHYSIOLOGY		
	Eyes	] Appetite Mechanism
	Mouth	] Digestive System
	Oesophagus	]
	Stomach	]
	Pyloric Sphincter	]
	Duodenum	]
	Jejenum	]
	Mammaries	] Hormonal System
	Ovaries, Testes	] Reproductive System
	Uterus	] Menstrual Cycle

PHYSICAL		
	Anaemia	Lactation Problems
	Appetite Disorders	Menstrual Cycle Disorders
	Belching	Nasal Problems
	Cold Sores	Poor Circulation- Lower Limbs
	Coldness in Digestive System	Ptosis - Visceral (ST)
	Colds & Flu	Pyrosis (Heartburn)
	Dry Complexion	Shoulder Pain
	Epigastric Discomfort	Stomach Problems/Ulcers
	Eye Problems	Thirst
	Halitosis (Bad Breath)	Toothache

PSYCHOLOGICAL		
	Affection	Maternal Issues
	Anxiety	Moody
	Burdened	Neurotic
	Compensatory Eating	Overactive
	Family (Relationships)	Overeating
	Frustration	Overthinking
	Future Orientated	Satisfaction
	Gullibility	Searching
	Hashing over Things	Stubborn ,
	Love	Unreliable

ZEN SHIATSU MERIDIAN CORRESPONDENCES

SPLEEN MERIDIAN
PI Ching

FACULTY		
	Spiritual Input	: YI, Thought
	Functions via	: Intelligence
	Represents	: Fertility
	Supplemented by	: Food & Intellectual Digestion
	Realised via	: Creating
	Dominant Zone	: Front
	Embryological Layer	: Mesoderm
	Meridian Nature	: Yin
	Tuning Time	: 9am - 11am

ANATOMY & PHYSIOLOGY		
	Cerebral Cortex	] Mento-Sensory Initiative
	Cerebrum	] Muscular System
	Muscles	]
	Lips	] Taste Mechanism
	Tongue	] Digestive System/
	Salivary Glands	] Enzymes
	Pancreas	]
	Gall Bladder	]
	Jejenum	]
	Mammaries	] Hormonal System
	Ovaries, Testes	] Reproductive System
	Uterus	]

PHYSICAL		
	Anaemia	Knee/Muscle Problems
	Appetite Disorders	Lack of Exercise
	Biliousness	Lack of Saliva
	Blood Disorders	Loose Stools
	Brownish Face	Memory Problems
	Craving Food/Liquids	Menstrual/Fertility Problems
	Digestive Disorders	Navel Stiffness
	Diabetes	Spinal Pain (Lower)
	Headaches	Sticky Dry Taste
	Heaviness in Limbs	Weight Problems

PSYCHOLOGICAL		
	Anguish	Overtechnical
	Anxiety	Overthinking
	Attention Seeking	Receptiveness
	Confidence	Restlessness
	Drowsy/Sleepiness	Self Pity
	Eating Habits	Stubborn
	Expressiveness	Support
	Home Life Issues (Family)	Timidity
	Intellectualisation	Worry
	Nervousness	Yearning (Maternal)

FUNCTIONAL SYSTEM	MERIDIAN / ORGAN FUNCTIONS IN ORIENTAL MEDICINE

ZANGFU	SPLEEN PI Governs transformation and transportation Controls the Blood (XUE) Controls the Muscles and Limbs Controls supportive Ki (maintains position of Organs) Opens into Mouth Manifests in the Lips Houses Thought (YI)	STOMACH WEI Controls reception, rotting and ripening of food and drink Controls transportation of food essences Controls descending Ki Origin of Fluids
IMAGE	The **Official** who transforms and transports the grain	The **Official** who controls the grain storehouses where the five tastes derive
CHINESE GOVT POST	**FINANCE MINISTER**	**TREASURY MINISTER**

ZEN SHIATSU	SPLEEN Meridian PI ching Governs secretion of digestive enzymes Reproductive hormones in relation to mammaries, ovaries, testes and uterus Promotes mental clarity	STOMACH Meridian WEI ching Governs the upper digestive tract through lips, oesophagus, stomach, and duodenum to the jejunum Controls appetite, lactation, ovarian, testicular and uterine function
BASIC	**Transforms and Transports Ki via Food and the Intellect**	**Receives Ki via Food and Drink**
SPECIFIC	**FOOD & INTELLECTUAL DIGESTION**	**INTAKE OF FOOD KI**
GENERAL	**NOURISHMENT**	

RESIDENTIAL TSUBO STUDIES

IDENTIFICATION	ACTION	INDICATIONS
ST 1 Chengqi CONTAINING TEARS Located directly inferior to the PUPIL on the inferior ridge of the ORBITAL CAVITY **** Moxibustion is contraindicated ****	Expels Wind (Int and Ext) Brightens the Eyes	Facial swelling, pain, conjunctivitis and paralysis of eyelid Redness, colour and night blindness Wasting of optic nerve
ST 3 Juliao BIG BONE Located directly inferior to ST 1 at the level of the inferior border of the ALA NASI	Expels Wind (Int and Ext) Relieves swelling Removes Channel obstructions	As ST 1 above Also facial paralysis and trigeminal neuralgia Nasal obstruction, toothache and lip pain
ST 9 Renying HUMAN'S WELCOME At the level of the LARYNGEAL prominence, located on the anterior border of the STERNOCLEIDOMASTOID muscle where the pulse of the COMMON CAROTID ARTERY can be felt SEA OF KI POINT ST & GB MEETING POINT **** Moxibustion is contraindicated **** **** Proceed with caution if blood pressure extremely high especially in early stages of cerebro vascular accident (CVA) ****	Regulates Ki and Blood Diffuses Lung Ki Benefits and moistens the Throat Stops pain Softens hard masses, resolves swellings	High or low blood pressure Hypertension Asthma, wheezing, belching, hiccup and nausea Oesophageal constriction with inability to swallow Sore throat, swollen larynx Acute obstruction of channels due to trauma (particularly lower back) Goitre (thyroid enlargement), pharyngitis (inflammation of rear cavity of the mouth) and tonsillitis

IDENTIFICATION	ACTION	INDICATIONS
ST 17 Ruzhong BREAST CENTRE Located in the centre of the NIPPLE in the 4th INTERCOSTAL SPACE (between the 4th and 5th RIBS), 4 SUN lateral to the Conception Vessel. ** **Acupuncture and Moxibustion contraindicated** ** ** **Breast Area contraindicated if cancer or inflammation are present** **	Mainly used as a reference point to locate tsubo in the Chest and Abdomen Insufficient Lactation ** Local tsubo Rugen, ST18, BREAST ROOT, is preferred for Breast problems, especially in women **	A method of promoting lactation by massage is outlined in P.212 of "Tsubo" by K. Serizawa Japan Publications, 1976
ST 25 Tianshu HEAVENLY AXIS 2 SUN lateral to the UMBILICUS, CV 8. BO or COLLECTING POINT of the LARGE INTESTINE	Regulates Intestinal functioning Relieves food retention Clears Heat (Intestines and Stomach)	Abdominal swelling, constipation, intestine pain Epigastric burning sensation, constipation, thirst, foul smelling loose stools or chronic diarrhoea, mental irritation
ST 34 Liangqiu CONNECTING MOUND Located 2 SUN superior to the lateral superior border of the PATELLA ACCUMULATING POINT	Regulates Stomach Ki Removes Channel obstructions Expels Dampness and Wind	Acid regurgitation, stomach ache and nausea, etc Lower limb pain Pain and swelling of knee and surrounding tissues
ST 36 Zusanli FOOT THREE MILES 3 SUN inferior to the lateral FORAMEN of the PATELLA (ST35), one finger breadth lateral to the anterior crest of the TIBIA. SEA POINT EARTH POINT	Tonifies Ki and Blood especially Stomach and Spleen Regulates nutritive and defensive Ki Expels Wind, Cold and Damp Raises Yang (use MOXA) ST 36 with CV 6 and GV 20 Regulates Intestines	Lack of vitality with weak muscle tone Lack of appetite, epigastric pain and poor digestion Anaemia Sweating after Wind Cold invasion Fatigue of extremities Oedema Aching muscles and joints Knee problems Prolapse of organs especially Stomach and Intestines Abdominal pain and distension, constipation and diarrhoea

IDENTIFICATION	ACTION	INDICATIONS
ST 40 Fenglong ABUNDANT BULGE 8 SUN inferior to the lateral FORAMEN of the PATELLA (ST35), two finger breadths lateral to the anterior crest of the TIBIA CONNECTING POINT	Resolves Damp and Phlegm Clears Stomach Heat Calms the Mind	Catarrh, phlegm as lumps/cysts Asthma, mental disturbances, muzzy or dizziness of the head Cloudy urine, mucus in stools Epigastric tightness and nervous anxiety Anxiety, fears and phobias due to lack of mental clarity
ST 42 Chongyang RUSHING YANG 1.3 SUN distal to ST 41 at the highest point of the DORSUM of the FOOT on the pulse of the DORSAL ARTERY SOURCE POINT	Tonifies Stomach and Spleen Calms the Mind Removes Channel obstructions	Lack of appetite, epigastric pain and distension, constipation Anxiety, hysteria and chronic restlessness Weakness, pain, swelling and muscular wasting (atrophy) of the foot Coldness in all joints Paralysis of lower extremities
ST 44 Neiting INNER COURTYARD 0.5 SUN proximal to the web margin between the 2nd and 3rd TOES SPRING POINT WATER POINT	Clears Heat Eliminates Wind from Face Stops pain Eliminates fullness	Bleeding gums, epigastric pain or burning sensation Heartburn Bleeding nose or gums Facial paralysis, trigeminal neuralgia Pain on stomach channel, particularly lower jaw, toothache Intestinal pain with fullness
ST 45 Lidui SPIRITS EXCHANGE About 0.1 SUN from the lateral corner of the 2nd TOENAIL WELL POINT METAL POINT	Calms the Mind Clears Heat and Damp Heat	Insomnia, hysteria, disorientation and dream disturbed sleep Indigestion, facial oedema, toothache, sore throat, bleeding nose and gums

IDENTIFICATION	ACTION	INDICATIONS
SP 1 Yinbai HIDDEN CLARITY About 0.1 SUN from the medial corner of the 1st TOENAIL WELL POINT WOOD POINT	Regulates Blood Strengthens the Spleen Calms the Mind	Stasis of blood in Uterus All types of bleeding due to Spleen deficiency including uterine, nasal, stomach, bladder or intestine bleeding Excessive dreaming, depression and mental restlessness
SP 3 Taibai GREAT BRIGHTNESS Located proximal and inferior to the head of the 1st METATARSAL bone at the junction of the red and white skin SOURCE POINT STREAM POINT EARTH POINT	Strengthens the Spleen Resolves Damp Strengthens and straightens the Spine	Tiredness due to excessive mental work Lack of mental clarity and memory lapses Loose stools and diarrhoea Confused thinking, muzzy head, stuffy chest No appetite, epigastric fullness, abdominal bloating, difficult urination, cloudy urine and vaginal discharge Retention of phlegm in Lungs Chronic backache
SP 6 Sanyinjiao THREE YIN MEETING Located 3 SUN directly superior to the vertex of the MEDIAL MALLEOLUS on the posterior border of the TIBIA MEETING POINT OF LIVER AND KIDNEY ON SPLEEN MERIDIAN ** Contraindicated in pregnancy **	Strengthens the Spleen Resolves Damp Smooths flow of Liver Ki Calms the Mind Tonifies Kidneys (Yin) Moves Blood Regulates Uterus and menstruation. Stops pain.	Tiredness, loose stools and poor appetite Chronic tiredness (c/w ST 36) Mucus in stools, urinary infection or pain, vaginal discharge Painful menstruation, abdominal pain, constipation Irritability and frustration, insomnia Dry mouth with thirst Dizziness, tinnitus and night sweats Painful menstruation with clotted blood, dark blood in stools Any gynaecological complaint Absence, excessive or painful menses, irregular menstrual cycle

IDENTIFICATION	ACTION	INDICATIONS
SP 9 Yinlingquan YIN MOUND SPRING Located on the inferior border of the MEDIAL CONDYLE of the TIBIA in a depression between the posterior border of the TIBIA and the GASTROCNEMIUS muscle 13 SUN proximal to the vertex of the MEDIAL MALLEOLUS SEA POINT WATER POINT	Resolves Dampness Benefits Lower Heater Removes Channel obstructions	Difficult urination, retention of urine, painful urination, cloudy urine Vaginal discharge, diarrhoea with foul smelling stools, oedema of the legs or abdomen Knee pain including swollen knee (Damp)
SP 10 Xuehai SEA OF BLOOD With the KNEE flexed located 2 SUN superior to the medial superior ridge of the PATELLA	Removes stasis of Blood Cools the Blood	Acute or chronic, painful or irregular menstruation Psoriasis, eczema and skin rashes of hot nature Uterine bleeding between menses or excessive menstrual bleeding
SP 21 Dabao GENERAL CONTROL Located in the 6th INTERCOSTAL SPACE on the mid axillary line midway between the AXILLA (HT 1) and the free end of the 11th RIB (LV 13) GENERAL CONNECTING POINT	Moves Blood in the blood connecting Channels	Muscular pain moving through body due to blood stasis

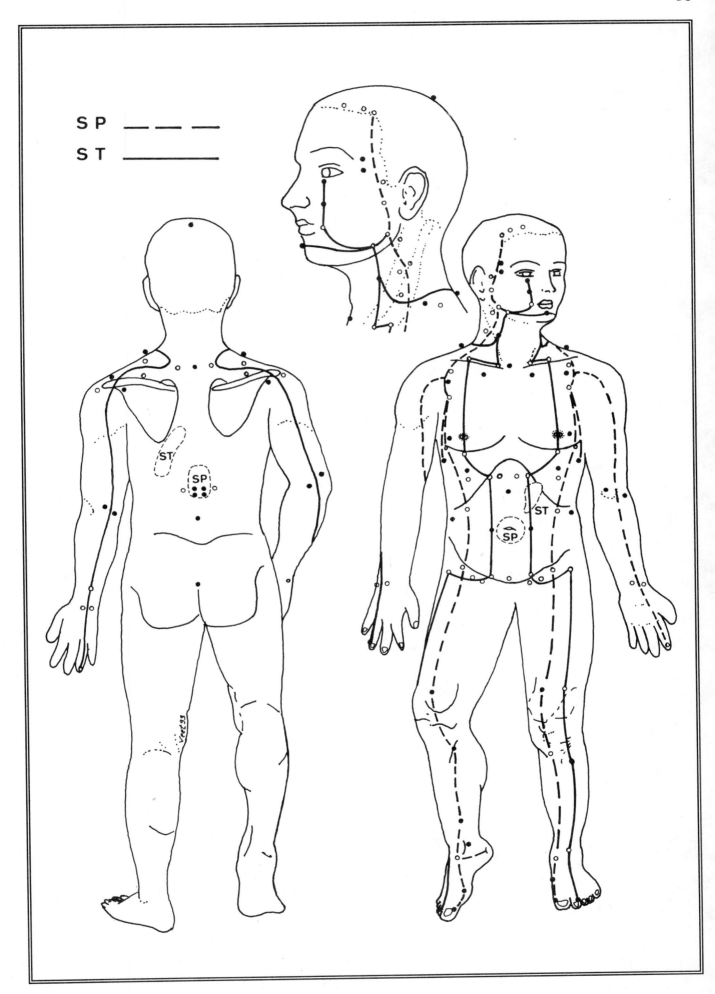

SP _ _ _ _

ST _____

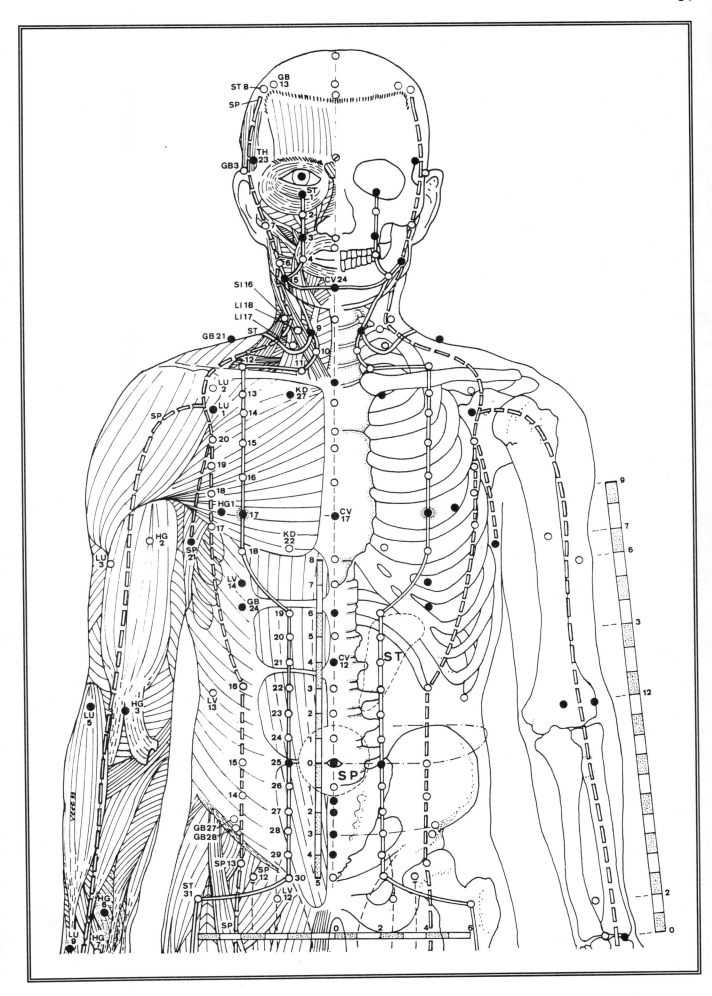

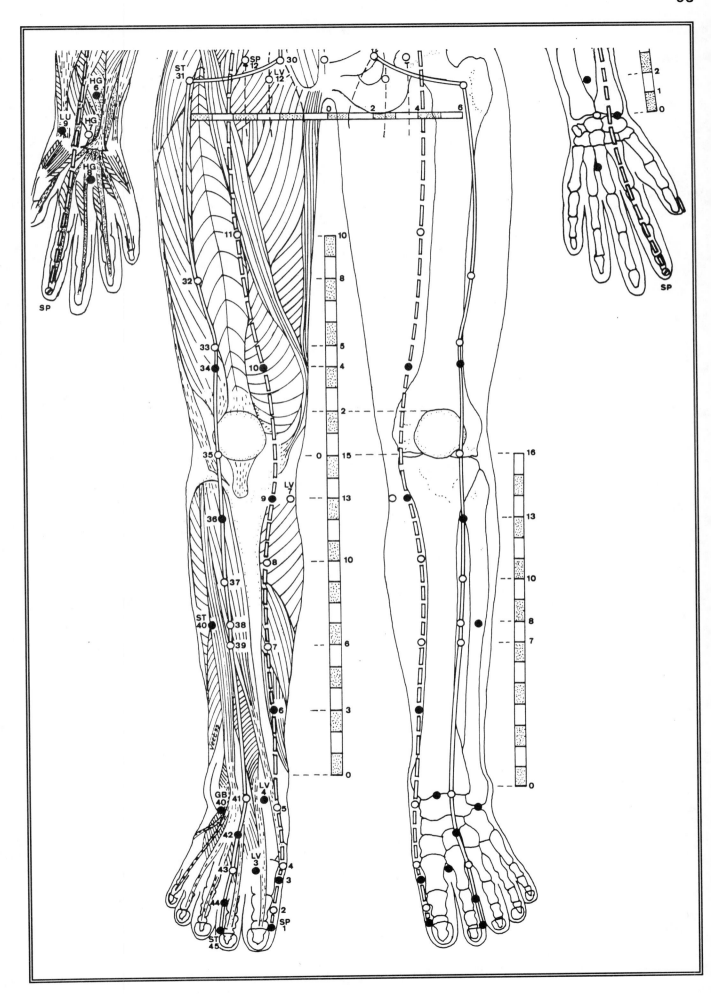

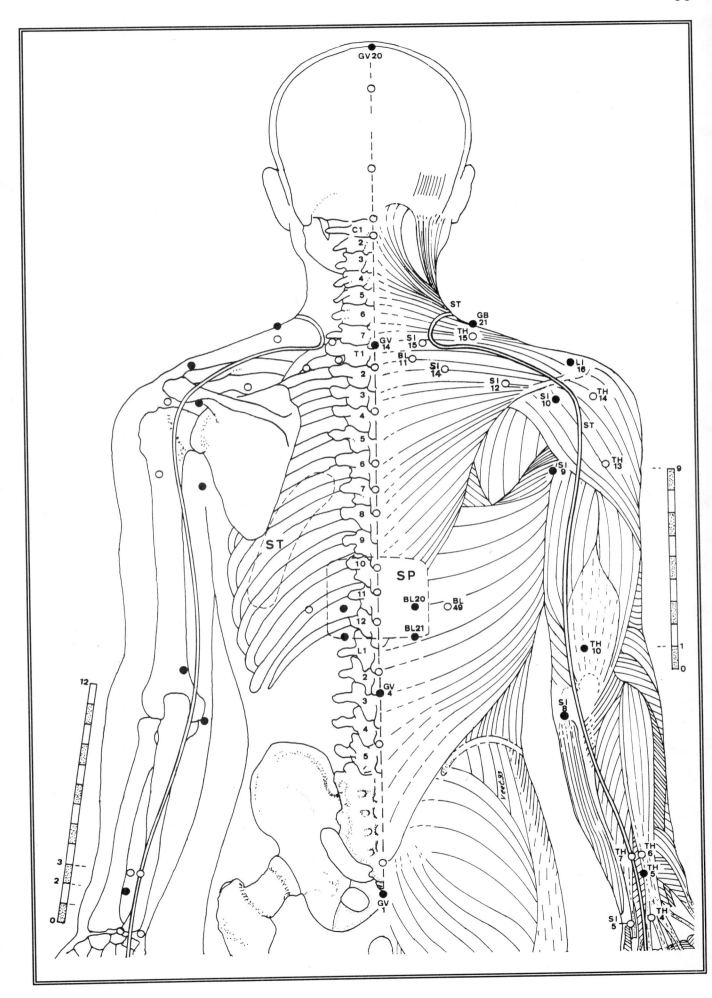

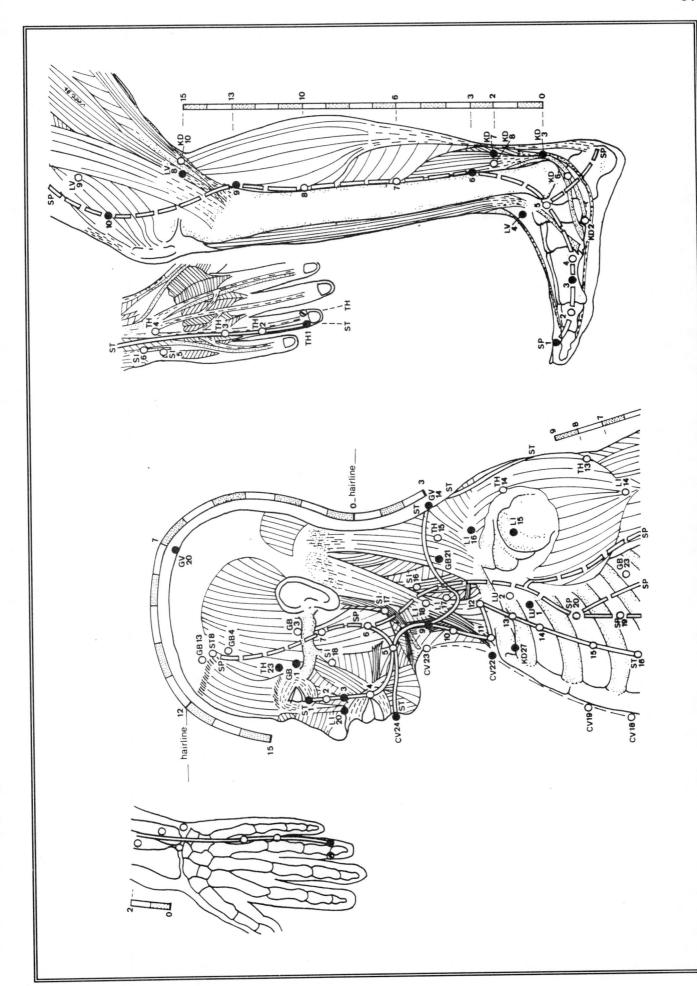

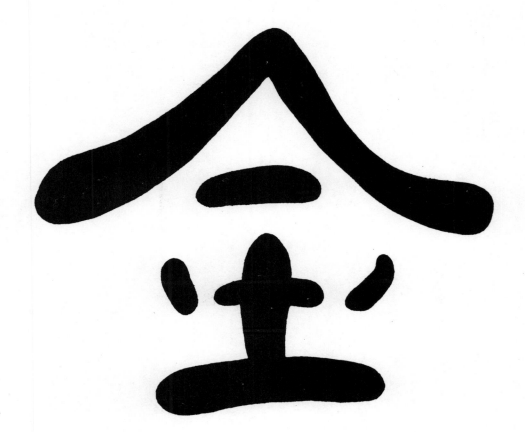

THE FIVE ELEMENT CORRESPONDENCES

FACULTY

Spiritual	Corporeal Soul
	PO
	Vitality
Genetic	Interaction
Cycle	Harvest
Yin/Yang	Lesser Yin
Quality	Solidified

ENVIRONMENTAL

Season	Autumn
Climate	Dry
Direction	West
Part of Day	Evening,
	7pm-12am
Colour	White

BODY

Organ	**Yin**	Lung
	Yang	Large Intestine
Tissue		Skin
Sense Organ		Nose
Senses		Smell
Branch		Body Hair
Skin Colour		White, Pale
Odour		Rotten
Fluid		Mucus

EMOTIONAL

Emotion	Grief
	Positivity
Sound, Voice	Weeping
	Wailing
Action	Coughing

FOOD

Animal	Horse
Fruit	Peach
Grain	Rice
Vegetable	Onion, Small &
	Contracted
Taste	Spicy

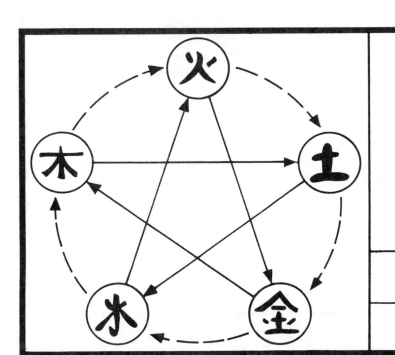

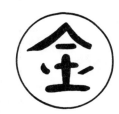

METAL

ZEN SHIATSU MERIDIAN CORRESPONDENCES

LUNG MERIDIAN
FEI ching

FACULTY		
	Spiritual Input	: PO, Corporeal Soul
	Functions via	: Physical Body
	Represents	: Structure
	Supplemented by	: Intake of Pure Ki
	Realised via	: Interacting
	Dominant Zone	: Outside
	Embryological Layer	: Ectoderm
	Meridian Nature	: Yin
	Tuning Time	: 3am - 5am

ANATOMY & PHYSIOLOGY		
	Nose	] Respiratory System
	Sinuses	]
	Pharynx	] Vocals
	Larynx	]
	Bronchials	] Related to Brain Functioning
	Lungs	]
	Intercostal Muscles	]
	Diaphragm	]
	Skin (Pores)	]

PHYSICAL		
	Asthma	Fever
	Bronchitis	Headaches
	Colds & Flu	Heavy Headiness
	Congestion of Nose/Chest	Loss of Voice
	Constipation	Pale Complexion
	Coughs	Respiratory Disease
	Dizziness	Stiff Thumb
	Dry Skin	Tight Intercostal Muscles
	Emphysema	Upper Back Pain
	Extreme Fatigue	White of Eyes, Dull

PSYCHOLOGICAL		
	Crying/Weeping	Pent Up Emotions
	Depression	Reclusive
	Hypersensitivity	Rigid Concepts
	Inability to Relax	Selfishness
	Jealousy	Shallow Breathing
	Lack of Clear Thinking	Sighing
	Melancholy	Social Problems
	Obsessed with Details	Unending Grief
	Organisational Problems	Unenthusiastic
	Overanxious	Worry

ZEN SHIATSU MERIDIAN CORRESPONDENCES

LARGE INTESTINE MERIDIAN
TA CHANG ching

FACULTY		
	Spiritual Input	: PO, via Lung Meridian
	Functions via	: Physical Body
	Represents	: Borders
	Supplemented by	: Elimination
	Realised via	: Clarifying
	Dominant Zone	: Outside
	Embryological Layer	: Ectoderm
	Meridian Nature	: Yang
	Tuning Time	: 5am - 7am

ANATOMY & PHYSIOLOGY		
	Nose]	Respiratory System
	Sinuses]	
	Mouth]	Digestive System
	Ileocaecal Valve]	Mucus Excretions/Secretions
	Large Intestine]	Bowel Movement
	Anal (Int & Ext) Sphincters]	
	Skin]	Integumentary System

PHYSICAL		
	Coldness in Lower Hara	Intestinal Disease
	Colds & Flu	Jaw Problems
	Constipation	Nasal Congestion
	Diarrhoea	Oedema
	Dislike of Exercise	Shoulder Pain
	Dull Vision	Skin Problems
	Epistaxis (Nose Bleeds)	Tonsillitis
	Haemorrhoids	Toothache
	Headaches	Stiff Index Finger
	Hip Problems	Stiffness in general

PSYCHOLOGICAL		
	Casualness	Overbearing Attitude
	Closed Off	Overdependence
	Easily Disappointed	Relationship Difficulties
	Holding on/Hoarding	Releasing/Letting Go
	Insecurity	Rigidity
	Lack of Expression	Social Problems
	Laziness	Stuckness
	No Enthusiasm	Territorial Issues
	No Initiative	Unhappiness
	Opinionated	Worthiness

FUNCTIONAL SYSTEM	MERIDIAN / ORGAN FUNCTIONS IN ORIENTAL MEDICINE

ZANGFU	LUNG	LARGE INTESTINE
	FEI	DA CHANG
	Governs Ki and Respiration Controls dispersing and descending Controls Channels and Blood Vessels Regulates Water Passages Controls Skin and Body Hair Opens into Nose Houses Corporeal Soul (PO)	Receives impure Material, absorbs Liquid and excretes the Stools
IMAGE	The **Minister** from whom policies are derived	The **Official** in charge of transmission
CHINESE GOVT POST	**PRIME MINISTER**	**FOREIGN MINISTER**

ZEN SHIATSU	LUNG Meridian	LARGE INTESTINE Meridian
	FEI ching	TA CHANG ching
	Governs Respiration via intake of Ki and elimination of Gases by exhalation Relates to regulation of Brain function and state of Mind	Elimination and excretion of waste material Harmonise emotions via appropriate hold on/let go response
BASIC	**Exchange of Gases via Respiration for Survival**	**Elimination of Processed Food and Emotive Ki**
SPECIFIC	**INTAKE OF PURE KI**	**ELIMINATION**
GENERAL	**VITALITY**	

RESIDENTIAL TSUBO STUDIES

IDENTIFICATION	ACTION	INDICATIONS
LU 1 Zhong Fu CENTRAL PALACE 1 SUN inferior to the centre of the INFRACLAVICULAR FOSSA and 6 SUN lateral to the Conception Vessel BO OR COLLECTING POINT FOR LUNGS MEETING POINT OF LUNG AND SPLEEN (GREATER YIN)	Regulates Lung Ki Stops Cough Clears Heat Stimulates descending of Lung Ki Fullness of Chest Stops pain	Asthma, bronchitis with cough and wheezing, breathing difficulties Painful throat, stagnation from phlegm or blood stasis Shoulder or upper back pain
LU 5 Chize CUBIT MARSH With ELBOW slightly flexed, located on the transverse CUBITAL crease on the RADIAL side of the TENDON of the BICEPS BRACHII muscle SEA POINT WATER POINT **** Use Moxibustion with caution ****	Clears Lung Heat Expels Phlegm (Hot and Cold) Relaxes Sinew	Asthma, bronchitis, cough, fever, thirst and yellow sputum Yellow or white sputum, chilliness Pain and swelling of elbow and arm Inability to raise arm to head
LU 7 Lieque BROKEN SEQUENCE 1.5 SUN above the transverse crease of the WRIST. Proximal to the STYLOID process of the RADIUS CONNECTING POINT LUNG	Stimulates descending and dispersal of Lung Ki Expels Exterior Wind (Cold/Hot) Opens Nose Benefits Bladder and Water Passages Assists Emotional Expression Balances Corporeal Soul	Asthma, cough Common cold, flu, stiff neck, headache Sinus problems, sneezing, runny nose and loss of sense of smell Oedema and urinary retention Suppression of feelings related to worry, grief, sadness etc Tense shoulders with shallow breathing

IDENTIFICATION	ACTION	INDICATIONS
LU 9 Tai Yuan GREAT ABYSS Located on the transverse crease of the WRIST, at the RADIAL side of the RADIAL ARTERY between the RADIUS and the SCAPHOID bones SOURCE POINT STREAM POINT EARTH POINT INFLUENTIAL POINT for BLOOD VESSELS	Tonifies Lung Ki and gathering Ki Resolves Phlegm Promotes Blood circulation Tonifies Heart Ki	Lack of vitality, chronic tiredness Cold hands with weak voice Dry cough Chronic cough with yellow sticky sputum Poor circulation, cold hands and feet, chilblains and varicose veins Breathless on exertion, palpitations
LU 11 Shaoshang LESSER METAL'S NOTE Located about 0.1 SUN from the RADIAL corner of the THUMBNAIL WELL POINT WOOD POINT	Expels Ext & Int Wind Promotes resuscitation	Sore throat, dry mouth High fever with sweating Loss of consciousness

IDENTIFICATION	ACTION	INDICATIONS
LI 1 Shang Yang METAL'S NOTE YANG Located about 0.1 SUN from the RADIAL corner of the 2nd FINGERNAIL WELL POINT METAL POINT **** Use Moxibustion with caution ****	Clears Heat Expels Wind and Cold Removes obstructions Revives consciousness	Sore throat, acute conjunctivitis Shoulder pain radiating to the Supraclavicular Fossa Loss of consciousness
LI 4 Hegu JOINING VALLEY On the back of the HAND, between the 1st and 2nd METACARPAL bones and about 0.5 SUN above the web margins slightly towards the INDEX FINGER SOURCE POINT **** Contraindicated during pregnancy ****	Expels Wind Heat Releases the Exterior Promotes descending of Lung Ki Stops pain Removes Channel obstructions Calms the Mind (roots Ki to Hara) Strengthens defensive Ki Promotes Labour	Nasal congestion, sneezing, burning eyes, hay fever Cough, stiff neck, aversion to cold Common cold and flu Intestinal and uterine pain Arm or shoulder pain, toothache, frontal headache, sinusitis, trigeminal neuralgia, facial paralysis Anxiety Asthma, bronchitis, cold etc Delayed or difficult labour
LI 10 Shousanli ARM THREE MILES Located 2 SUN distal to LI 11 on a line connecting to LI 5	Removes Channel obstructions Tonifies Ki	Any muscular problem affecting the arm and hands Wasting of arm muscles Sluggish intestines, lack of vitality (especially upper body)

IDENTIFICATION	ACTION	INDICATIONS
LI 11 Quchi CROOKED POND With the ELBOW flexed, located between the lateral end of the transverse CUBITAL crease and the LATERAL EPICONDYLE of the HUMERUS SEA POINT EARTH POINT	Expels Exterior Wind Heat Clears Heat Cools Blood Clears Damp Heat Removes Channel obstructions Benefits the Sinews	Fever, chills, stiff neck, sweating, runny nose and body aches Eczema, psoriasis, urticaria (nettle rash) Skin eruptions (acne), cystitis, urethritis, heavy feeling, loose stools, abdominal distension Goitre (thyroid swelling) Muscular wasting (atrophy) Pain and paralysis of arm and shoulders Rheumatism and arthritis
LI 15 Jianyu SHOULDER'S CORNER Located directly inferior to the anterior border of the ACROMION where a depression is formed when the ARM is abducted	Removes Channel obstructions Benefits Sinews Stops Shoulder pain Expels Wind and clears Heat	Frozen shoulder Shoulder bursitis (inflammation), pain or stiffness Atrophy (wasting) of upper limbs Muscular spasms Paralysis of arm Urticaria (nettle rash) due to Wind-Heat Excessive sweating
LI 16 Jugu GREAT BONE Located in the depression between the ACROMION extremity of the CLAVICLE and the SCAPULAR SPINE	Removes Channel obstructions Opens Chest Stimulates descending of Lung Ki Subdues ascending rebellious Ki	Frozen shoulder Inflammation, pain and stiffness of shoulder and upper back zone Asthma, breathlessness and cough Hypertension
LI 20 Ying Xiang WELCOME FRAGRANCE Located on the NASOLABIAL SULCUS, level with the mid point of the lateral border of the ALA NASI MEETING POINT STOMACH AND LARGE INTESTINE	Dispels Exterior Wind	All nose problems, sneezing, loss of sense of smell, bleeding nose, runny nose, stuffy nose, allergic rhinitis (nasal inflammation), sinusitis

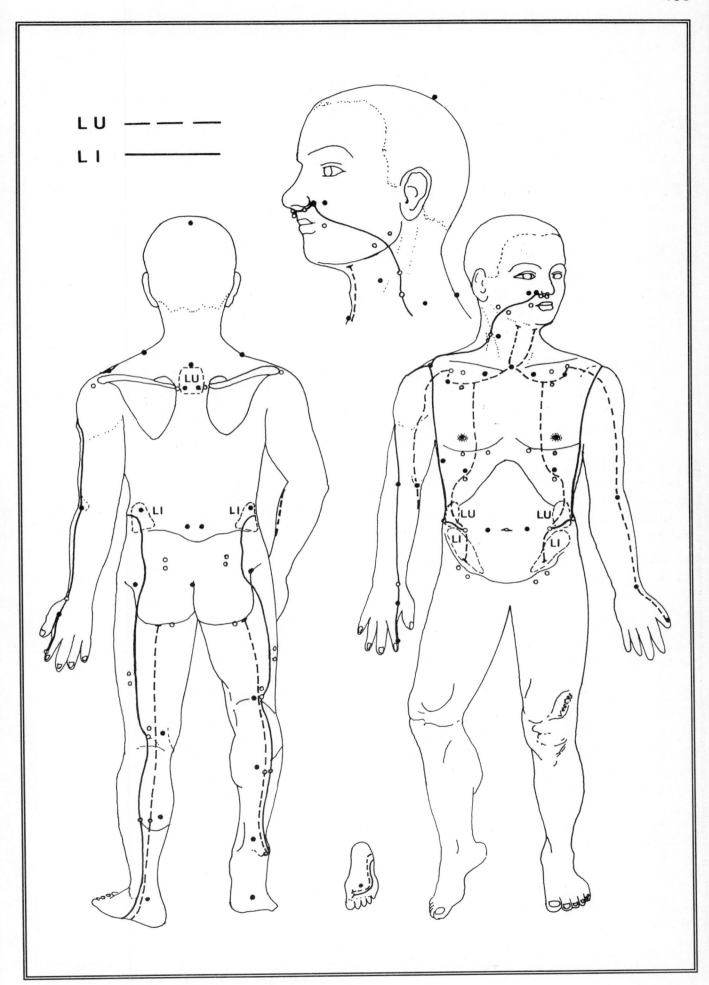

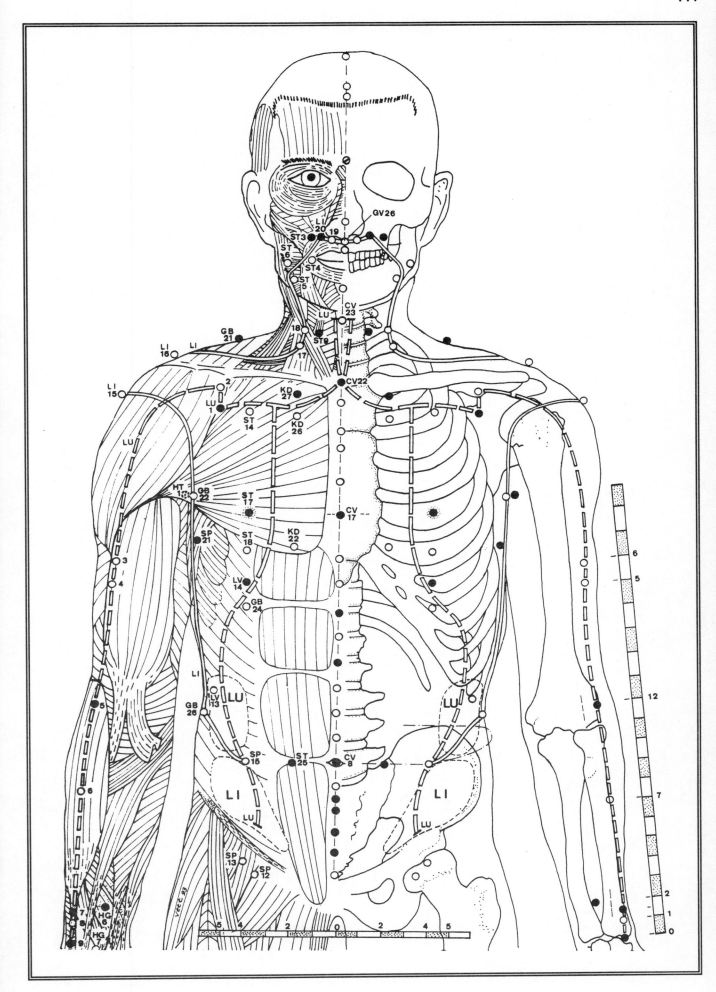

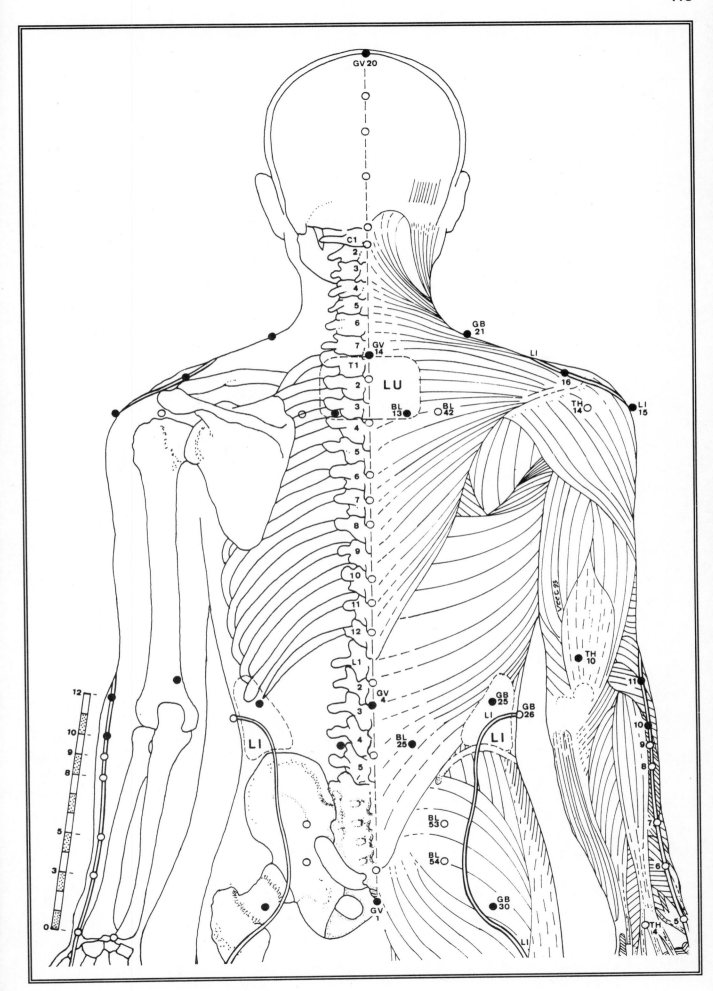

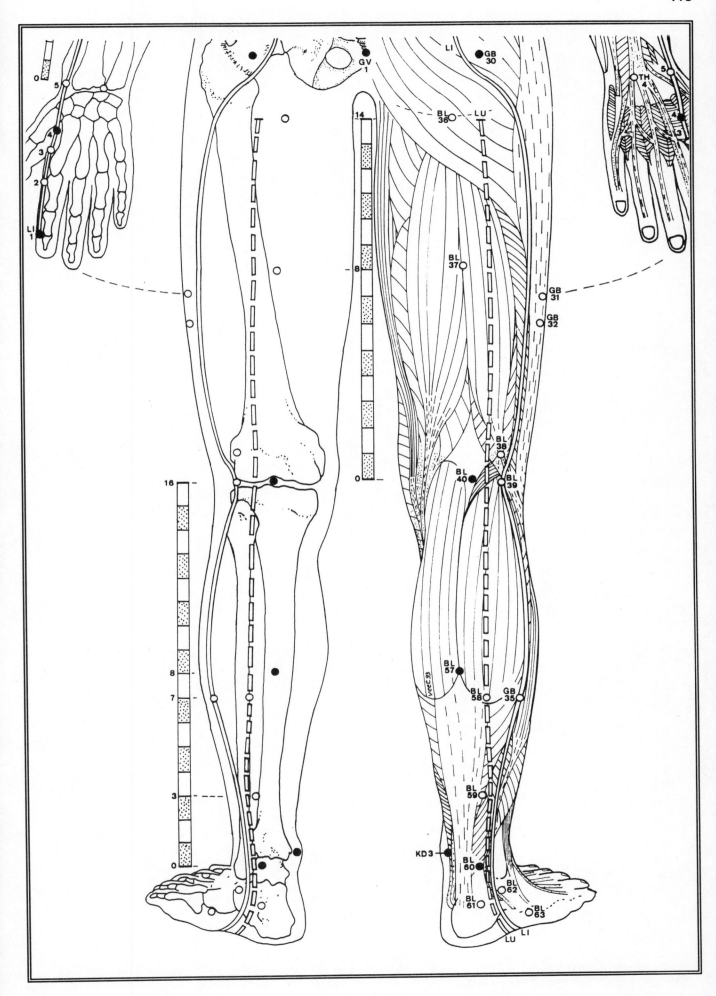

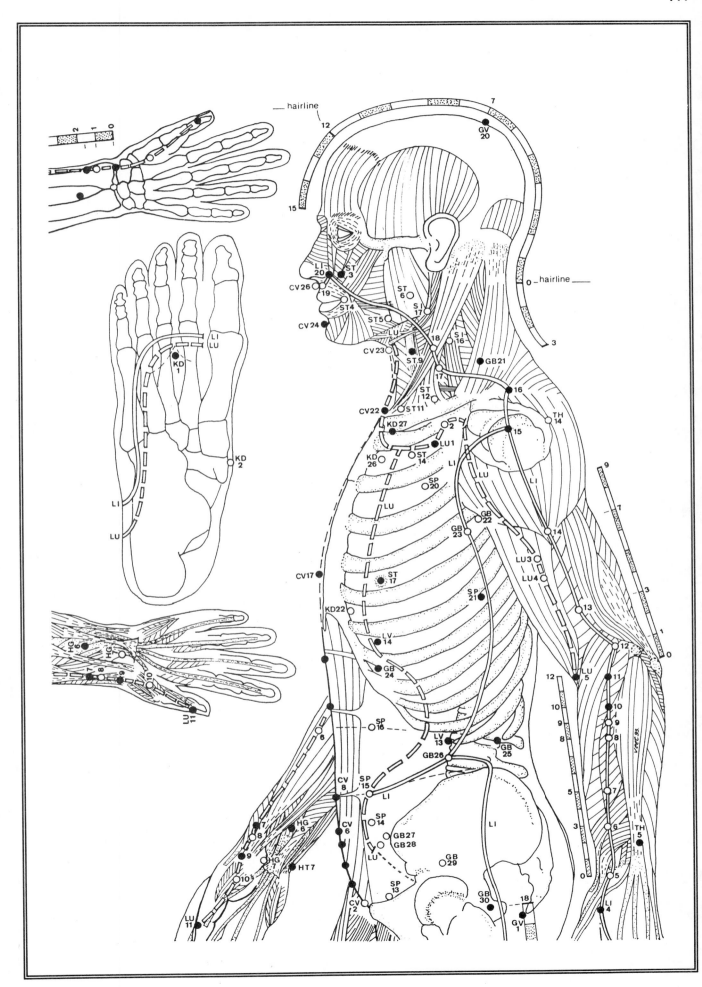

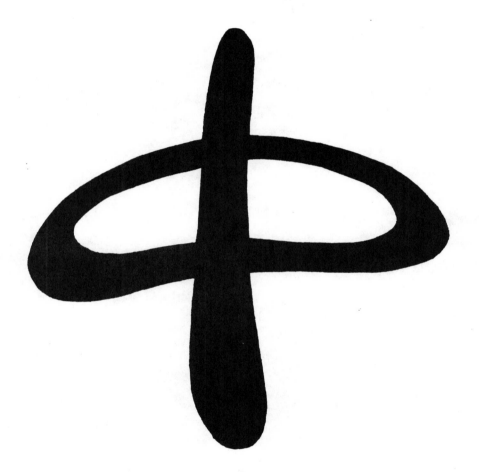

IDENTIFICATION	ACTION	INDICATIONS
CV 1 Huiyin MEETING OF YIN Located at the centre of the PERINEUM between the ANUS and the SCROTUM in males, and between the ANUS and POSTERIOR LABIAL COMMISSURE in females. CONNECTING POINT	Nourishes Yin Stabilises Essence Resolves Damp Heat Restores consciousness	Incontinence, reproductive disorders Genital or perineal pain, itching or swelling Cessation of breathing due to near drowning
CV 3 Zhongji CENTRAL POLE 4 SUN inferior to the UMBILICUS on the anterior midline BO or COLLECTING POINT for BLADDER CV, SP, LIV, KD MEETING POINT **** Contraindicated during pregnancy ****	Regulates Bladder Resolves Damp Heat Clears Heat	Urinary incontinence or retention Pain and burning on urination, inflammation of Bladder (Cystitis) Genital pain or itching Blood in urine, burning urination
CV 4 Guanyuan GATE TO THE ORIGINAL KI 3 SUN inferior to the UMBILICUS on the anterior midline BO or COLLECTING POINT for the SMALL INTESTINE GV, SP, LIV, KD MEETING POINT **** Contraindicated in pregnancy ****	Nourishes Blood and Yin Regulates the Uterus Tonifies the Kidneys Benefits Original Ki Tonifies Yang (with Moxibustion) Regulates Small Intestine Roots Ethereal Soul	Severe anxiety, absence or scanty menstruation and uterine disorders Asthma, urinary disorders due to chronic fatigue or constitutional weakness Chronic fatigue or weakness with cold extremities Diarrhoea Vague feeling of fear at night

IDENTIFICATION	ACTION	INDICATIONS
CV 5 Shimen STONE GATE 2 SUN inferior to the UMBILICUS on the anterior midline BO or COLLECTING POINT for the TRIPLE HEATER **** Contraindicated in pregnancy ****	Tonifies Original Ki Regulates fluids in Lower Heater	Kidney deficiency, poor constitution Abdominal oedema, urinary retention or incontinence Diarrhoea or vaginal discharge
CV 6 Qihai SEA OF KI 1.5 SUN inferior to the UMBILICUS on the anterior midline **** Contraindicated in Pregnancy ****	Tonifies Ki and Yang (c/w Moxibustion) Tonifies Original Ki (c/w Moxibustion) Resolves Dampness (Lower Heater) Regulates Ki	Extreme physical and mental exhaustion and depression Fatigue, loose stools, chills, abundant pale urination, depression and lack of willpower Vaginal discharge or loose stools with mucus, difficult urination Stagnancy, pain or distension in the lower abdomen
CV 8 Shenque SPIRITS PALACE GATE Located in the centre of the UMBILICUS. **** Acupuncture contraindicated ****	Tonifies Yang Tonifies and strengthens the Spleen (Use with indirect Moxibustion after filling Umbilicus with salt)	Extreme fatigue and internal cold Chronic diarrhoea
CV 12 Zhongwan MIDDLE STOMACH CAVITY 4 SUN superior to the UMBILICUS on the anterior midline BO or COLLECTING POINT for the STOMACH GATHERING POINT for YANG ORGANS FRONT COLLECTING POINT of the MIDDLE HEATER	Tonifies Stomach and Spleen (c/w Moxibustion for Cold) Resolves Dampness	Lack of appetite, digestive weakness, tiredness with cold Abdominal distension and pain Constipation with headache General feeling of heaviness

IDENTIFICATION	ACTION	INDICATIONS
CV 14 Juque GREAT PALACE 6 SUN superior to the UMBILICUS on the anterior midline BO or COLLECTING POINT for the HEART	Subdues rebellious Stomach Ki Calms the Mind Clears the Heart	Mental anxiety, heartburn, vomiting, regurgitation, hiccups, difficulty in swallowing (mainly due to emotional origin) Forgetfulness, fearful palpitations, anxiety
CV 17 Shanzhong or Tanzhong CENTRAL ALTAR Located between the NIPPLES, level with the 4th INTERCOSTAL SPACE on the anterior midline BO or COLLECTING POINT for the HEART GOVERNOR GATHERING POINT for KI SEA OF KI POINT FRONT COLLECTING POINT for UPPER HEATER	Tonifies Ki Regulates Ki Resolves Phlegm Facilitates Lactation	Breathlessness, bronchitis, asthma, lack of vitality with pale face, cough, chest pain, palpitations, intercostal neuralgia, hiccups, anxiety Cough, chronic bronchitis Insufficient lactation
CV 22 Tiantu HEAVENS CHIMNEY Located at the SUPRASTERNAL FOSSA 0.5 SUN above the STERNAL NOTCH	Descends Lung Ki Resolves Phlegm Clears Heat	Acute and chronic asthma and cough Acute bronchitis with profuse sputum, lung and throat mucus Sore throat due to exterior pathogen (Wind-Heat)
CV 24 Chengjiang SALIVA RECEIVER Located in the depression inferior to the MENTOLABIAL GROOVE on the anterior midline CV, GV, ST & LI MEETING POINT	Expels Exterior Wind	Paralysis of the face and mouth

RESIDENTIAL TSUBO STUDIES

IDENTIFICATION	ACTION	INDICATIONS
GV 1 Changqiang LASTING STRENGTH Located midway between the tip of the COCCYX and the ANUS CONNECTING POINT GV, KD & GB MEETING POINT	Regulates the GV & CV Resolves Damp Heat Calms the Mind	Back pain, fatigue Haemorrhoids Hysteria, hypomania
GV 4 Mingmen GATE OF LIFE Located inferior to the spinous process of the 2nd LUMBAR VERTEBRA on the posterior midline	Tonifies Kidney Yang (c/w Moxibustion) (caution if Heat symptoms anywhere) Nourishes Original Ki Benefits Essence Strengthens Lower Back Expels Cold (Yang deficiency)	Fatigue, chilliness, abundant clear urination, depression, weakness of legs, pale tongue. Chronic physical and mental weakness, reproductive disorders. Chronic lumbar stiffness or pain. Chronic diarrhoea, intestinal pain, incontinence, reproductive disorders.
GV 14 Dazhui BIG VERTEBRA Located inferior to the spinous process of the 7th CERVICAL VERTEBRA on the posterior midline GV, BL, GB & ST MEETING POINT SEA OF KI POINT	Releases the Exterior Expels Wind Clears Heat Regulates Nutritive and Defensive Ki Calms the Mind Stimulates the Brain	Asthma, common cold, fullness of chest. Neck and spinal stiffness and pain. Fever and chills. Epilepsy Hay Fever and Eczema, sweating Mania, hysteria, headache. Unclear thinking.

IDENTIFICATION	ACTION	INDICATIONS
GV 20 Baihui HUNDRED MEETINGS Located on the midline of the HEAD, halfway between the frontal hairline and the vertex of the EXTERNAL OCCIPITAL PROTUBERANCE (INION) MEETING POINT of all the YANG CHANNELS SEA OF MARROW POINT **** Moxibustion contraindicated if high blood pressure or heat symptoms ****	Calms the Mind Tonifies Yang (c/w Moxibustion) Strengthens Spleen ascending function Promotes resuscitation c/w GV26 & HG6	Unclear thinking, depression Prolapse of Stomach, Bladder, Uterus, Anus or Vagina. Haemorrhoids Unconsciousness
GV 26 Renzhong MIDDLE OF PERSON Located on the PHILTRUM about one third the distance from the base of the NOSE to the tip of the LIP **** Moxibustion is contraindicated **** GV, LI, ST MEETING POINT	Promotes resuscitation Benefits Lumbar Spine	Unconsciousness, drowsiness Acute lower back sprain
GV 28 Yinjiao GUMS CROSSING Located between the upper LIP and the upper GUM in the LABIAL FRENUM CONNECTING POINT for GV and CV	Resolves Damp Heat	Painful, swollen gums, Haemorrhoids

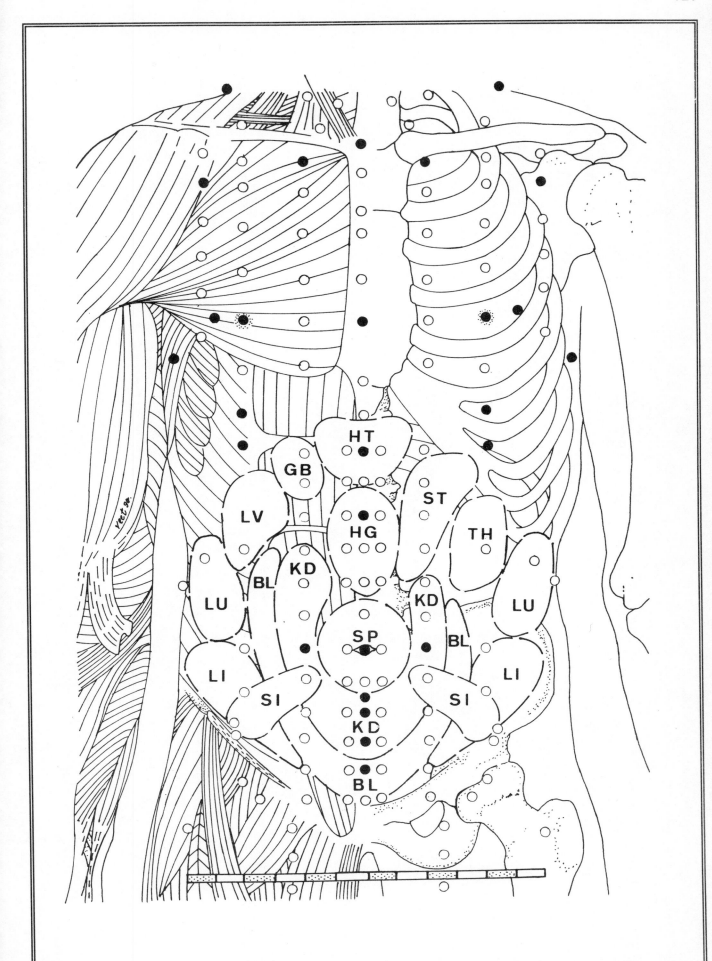

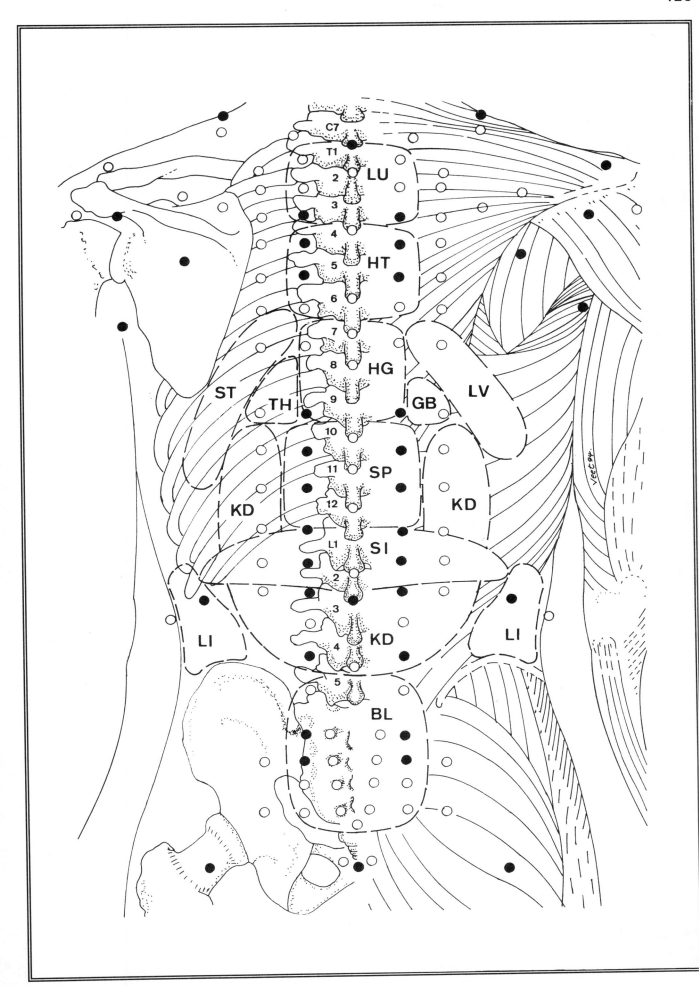

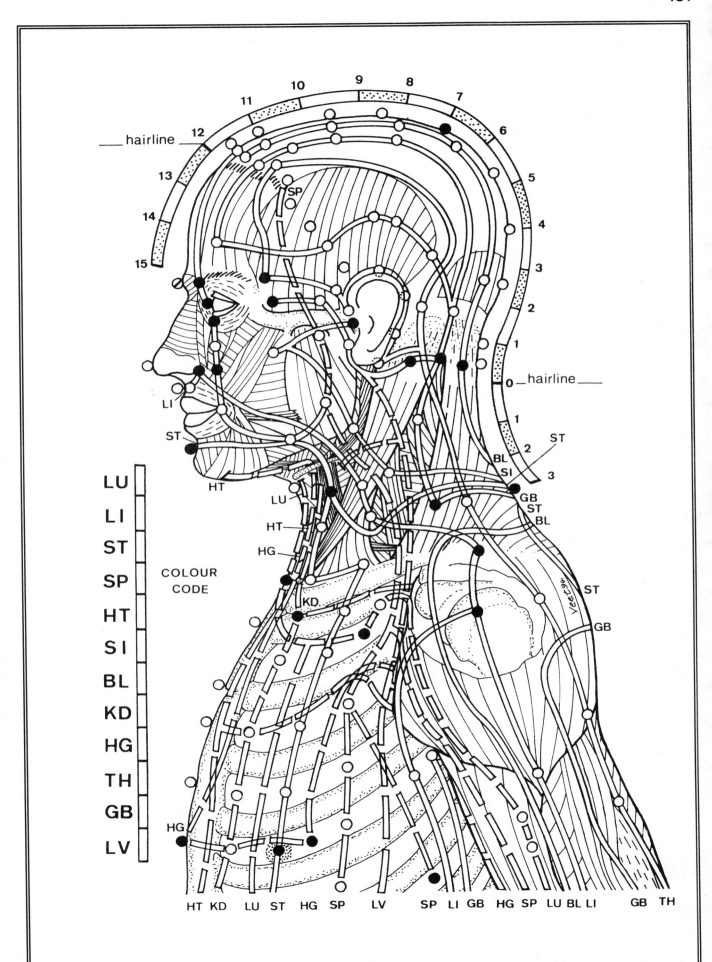

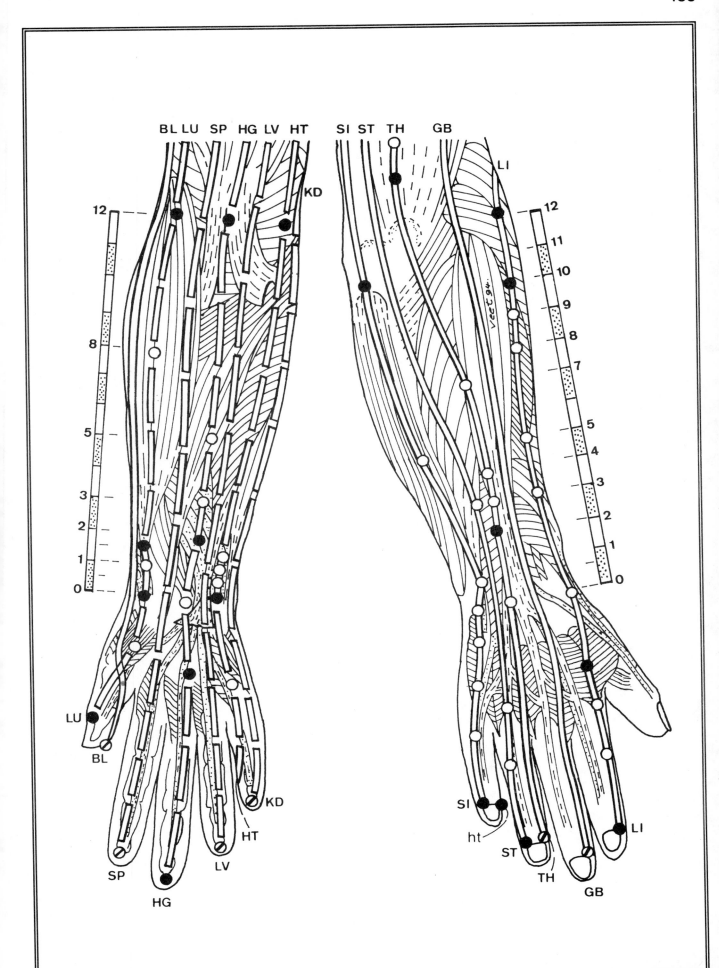

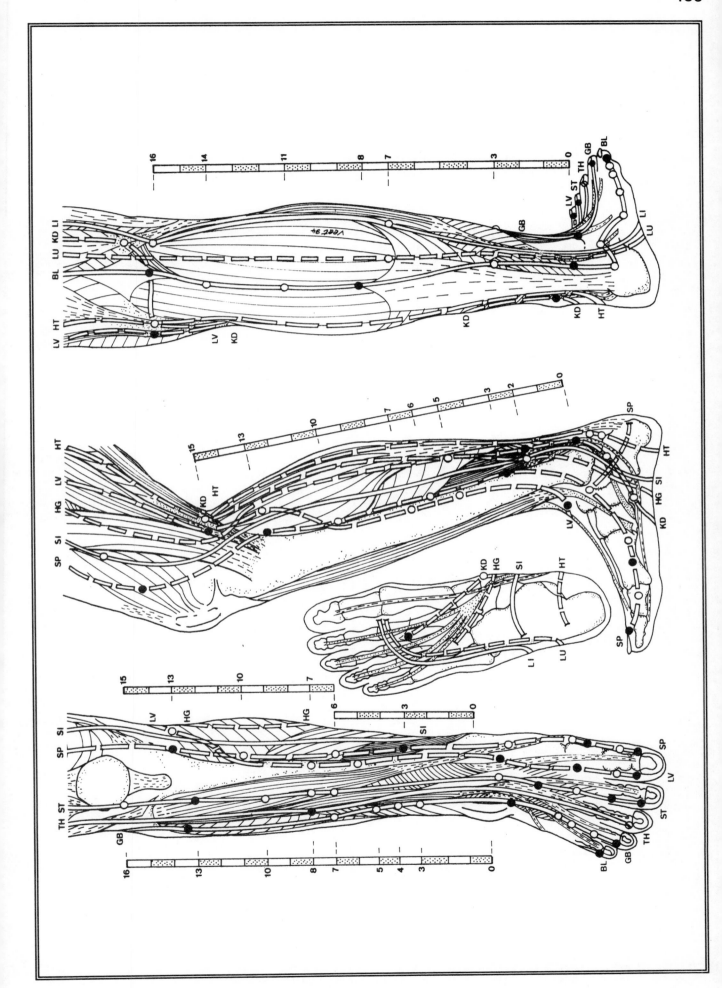

BIBLIOGRAPHY AND REFERENCES

Blakey P. The Muscle Book, Stafford : Bibliotek Books, 1992

Brennan, B.A. Hands of Light. New York : Bantam Books, 1988

Chaitow, L. Osteopathic Self Treatment. London : Diamond Books, 1993.

Chia, M. Chi Nei Tsang : Internal Organs Chi Massage. Huntington, N.Y, 1991

Connelly, D.M. Traditional Acupuncture : The Law of the Five Elements. Columbia : Trad. AC Centre, 1979

Dawes, N. The Shiatsu Workbook : A Beginners Guide. London : Piatkus, 1991

Fundamentals of Chinese Acupuncture (An Outline of Chinese Acupuncture). The Academy of Traditional Chinese Medicine. Peking : Indian edition, Bombay : Taraporevala & Sons, 1988

Hashimoto, K. MD with Kawakami, Y. Sotai, Balance and Health through Natural Movement. Tokyo : Japan Publications Inc., 1983

Hashimoto, K. Sotai : Natural Exercise. Oroville C.A. : George Ohsawa Macrobiotic Foundation, 1981

Jarmey, C. and Mojay, G. Shiatsu : The Complete Guide. London : Thorsons, 1991

Journal of Chinese Medicine Nos 33-44. Hove : TCM, 1990-1994.

Kapit, W. and Elson, L.M. The Anatomy Colouring Book. New York : Harper Collins, 1987

Kaptchuk, T.J. Chinese Medicine : The Web that has no Weaver. London : Century Hutchinson, 1983

Kenyon, J.N. 21st Century Medicine : A Layman's Guide to the Medicine of the Future. Wellingborough : Thorsons, 1986.

Kushi, M. How to see Your Health, Book of Oriental Diagnosis. Tokyo, New York : Japan Publications Inc, 1986

Lade, A. Acupuncture Points, Images and Functions. Seattle, USA : Eastland Press, 1989

Maciocia, G. The Foundations of Chinese Medicine. Edinburgh, London, Melbourne, New York : Churchill Livingstone, 1989

Maciocia, G. Tongue Diagnosis in Chinese Medicine. Seattle, USA : Eastland Press, 1987

Masunaga, S. Shiatsu Meridian Chart; Diagnosis and Treatment. Tokyo : Iokai Shiatsu Centre, 1970

Masunaga, S. Zen Imagery Exercises; Meridian Exercises for Wholesome Living. Tokyo, New York : Japan Publications Inc, 1987

Masunaga, S. with Ohashi, W. Zen Shiatsu; How to Harmonize Yin and Yang for Better Health. Tokyo, New York : Japan Publications Inc, 1977

Matsumoto, K and Birch, S. Hara Diagnosis; Reflections on the Sea. Brookline MA : Paradigm Publications, 1988

The Newest Illustrations of Acupuncture Points. Hong Kong: Medicine and Health Publishing Co, no date

Ohashi, W. Do It Yourself Shiatsu : How to Perform the Ancient Japanese Art of Acupuncture without needles. London : Unwin Hyman, 1979

Passmore, R. and Robson, J.S. eds. A Companion to Medical Studies, Vol 1, Anatomy, biochemistry, physiology and related subjects. Oxford, London, Edinburgh, Melbourne : Blackwell Scientific Publications, 1976

Pauchet, V. and Dupret, S. Pocket Atlas of Anatomy. Oxford : Oxford University Press, 1937

Prudden, B. Myotherapy; Complete Guide to Pain Free Living. New York : Ballantine Books, 1985.

Raynes, J. Figure Drawing and Anatomy for the Artist. London : Chancellor Press, 1993

Rofidal, J. Do-In : Eastern Massage and Yoga Techniques. Wellingborough : Thorsons 1981

Roper, N. ed. Pocket Medical Dictionary. Edinburgh, London, Melbourne and New York : Churchill Livingstone, 1987

Sasaki, P. and Andrews, C. Zen Shiatsu Residential Workshops, held at Grimstone Manor, Horrabridge 1989-91

Seem, M. Bodymind Energetics ; Towards a Dynamic Model of Health. Wellingborough : Thorsons, 1987

Sergel, D. The Macrobiotic Way of Zen Shiatsu. Tokyo and New York : Japan Publications Inc, 1989

Serizawa, K. Tsubo : Vital Points for Oriental Therapy. Tokyo and New York : Japan Publications Inc, 1976

Stanway, Dr. A. Prevention is Better @ An A-Z of Common Illnesses and Problems and How to Prevent Then. London, Melbourne, Auckland, Johannesburg: Century Hutchinson, 1986

Upledger, J. and Vredevoogd, J.D. Craniosacral Therapy. Seattle, WA : Eastland Press, 1983.

The Visual Dictionary of the Human Body. Various. London, New York, Stuttgart : Dorling Kindersley, 1991

Williams, J.C.P. Injury in Sport; Diagnostic Picture Tests. London : Wolfe Medical Publications, 1988

Wilson, K.J.W. Anatomy and Physiology in Health and Illness. Edinburgh, London, Melbourne and New York: Churchill Livingstone, 1987

Worsley, J.R. The Meridians of Chi Energy. Leamington Spa : The Collage of Traditional Chinese Acupuncture, 1985

Yang Jiason, Prof. The Way to Locate Acu-Points. Peking : Foreign Language Press, 1988